Praise for

"In their brilliant and highly accessible book, Stephen Porges and Karen Onderko demonstrate how deeply understanding physiological and biological processes can lead to profound changes in mental health care delivery. Music, from didgeridoo to Indian ragas, and from Mozart to Aretha Franklin, has always been a source of solace and restoration. But the Safe and Sound Protocol enhances this further by applying filters to the mosaic of sounds that provide just the optimal experience to restore both focus and peace of mind."

Bessel van der Kolk, MD
researcher, educator, and *New York Times*
bestselling author of *The Body Keeps the Score*

"I recently had the privilege of briefly trying the Safe and Sound Protocol described in this exciting new book and found the experience to be as advertised. I felt a shift toward more calm and openness. Using my language, it seems like the music helps protective parts relax so people can access more Self—that healing essence within everyone. I look forward to combining it with the approach I developed called Internal Family Systems, particularly with highly protective systems."

Richard C. Schwartz, PhD
American systemic family therapist and author of *No
Bad Parts* and *You Are the One You've Been Waiting For*

"This accessibly written book, grounded in Polyvagal Theory, uses inspiring case stories to show how sound attuned to human speech can help rebalance the nervous system, offering a powerful remedy for trauma and dysregulation."

David Drew Pinsky, MD
internist, addiction medicine specialist, television host,
and *New York Times* bestselling author of *The Mirror Effect*

"Porges and Onderko show significant potential for the Safe and Sound Protocol in addressing trauma-related disembodiment and Parkinson's disease. Their work paves the way for future research exploring sensory-based interventions across a variety of conditions."

Ruth A. Lanius, MD, PhD
professor of psychiatry and Harris-Woodman Chair in Mind-Body Medicine at the University of Western Ontario, Canada

"This book is a most welcome and informative guide to the theory, evidence base, and range of applications of the Safe and Sound Protocol. The combination of case studies and application of theory to real life scenarios breathes life into the implementation process, which will be invaluable to existing Safe and Sound Protocol practitioners and those exploring the use of the program for the first time."

Billy Smallwood, clinical director, and
Waveney Patel, clinical regional director
Witherslack Group UK

Safe
and
Sound

Also by Stephen W. Porges

*The Polyvagal Theory: Neurophysiological Foundations of
Emotions, Attachment, Communication, and Self-Regulation*

*The Pocket Guide to the Polyvagal Theory:
The Transformative Power of Feeling Safe*

*Clinical Applications of the Polyvagal Theory: The
Emergence of Polyvagal-Informed Therapies* (coeditor)

Polyvagal Safety: Attachment, Communication, Self-Regulation

Our Polyvagal World: How Safety and Trauma Change Us

Polyvagal Perspectives: Interventions, Practices, and Strategies

Safe and Sound

A Polyvagal Approach for Connection, Change, and Healing

Stephen W. Porges, PhD
Karen Onderko

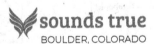

sounds true
BOULDER, COLORADO

Sounds True
Boulder, CO

Foreword © 2025 Peter Levine

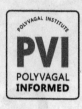

This book is not intended as a substitute for the medical recommendations of physicians, mental health professionals, or other health-care providers. Rather, it is intended to offer information to help the reader cooperate with physicians, mental health professionals, and health-care providers in a mutual quest for optimal well-being. We advise readers to carefully review and understand the ideas presented and to seek the advice of a qualified professional before attempting to use them.

Some names and identifying details have been changed to protect the privacy of individuals.

Published 2025

Cover design by Jess Morphew
Jacket design by Rachael Murray
Book design by Meredith Jarrett
Illustrations by Lisa Gleeson

Printed in the United States of America

BK06874

Library of Congress Cataloging-in-Publication Data

Names: Porges, Stephen W., author. | Onderko, Karen, author.
Title: Safe and sound : a polyvagal approach for connection, change, and healing / Stephen W. Porges and Karen Onderko.
Other titles: Polyvagal approach for connection, change, and healing
Description: Boulder, CO : Sounds True, 2025. | Includes bibliographical references and index.
Identifiers: LCCN 2024039618 (print) | LCCN 2024039619 (ebook) | ISBN 9781649632340 (paperback) | ISBN 9781649632357 (ebook)
Subjects: LCSH: Neuropsychiatry--Case studies. | Autonomic nervous system. | Affective neuroscience. | Mental illness--Treatment.
Classification: LCC RC341 .P78 2025 (print) | LCC RC341 (ebook) | DDC 616.80072/3--dc23/eng/20250116
LC record available at https://lccn.loc.gov/2024039618
LC ebook record available at https://lccn.loc.gov/2024039619

To SSP providers, past, present, and future:
By supporting client safety, you are the heart of SSP's effectiveness.

Contents

List of Tips and Practices

This list contains practical exercises to reset and rebalance the autonomic nervous system (ANS) that you can try on your own or with a friend.

Foreword

Learning how to create an environment that feels safe can help both clients and individuals in everyday situations reduce defensiveness, leading to deeper connections and greater understanding. With that in mind, it can be important to ask the questions *How often does therapy falter due to a client's defensiveness?* and *Do we really understand the nature of these defenses?* This understanding is crucial not only for therapists but also for anyone pursuing personal growth or navigating interpersonal relationships. By recognizing our own defensive patterns, we can foster healthier communication with others.

It is here that the polyvagal theory offers a fresh perspective, and the Safe and Sound Protocol (SSP) provides a renewed approach to finding such solutions. Through a detailed exploration of the theoretical underpinnings and practical applications of Polyvagal Theory and SSP, this book aims to enrich the reader's understanding of the fundamental nature of human defense mechanisms and the quest for psychological safety. It is a vital resource for anyone interested in enhancing the efficacy of therapeutic interventions or developing a compassionate approach to self-healing.

Polyvagal theory emphasizes the crucial role that the muscles of the face and head play in shaping how we perceive and respond to the world around us. It has provided the missing link, explaining how our biobehavioral state—whether we feel calm and connected, activated, or shutdown and dissociated—directly influences our perceptions and reactions to our environment and to others.

This is where the SSP comes in. It offers an effective solution to create the *physiological underpinning of safety*, which facilitates the formation of a therapeutic alliance and helps address underlying trauma. By focusing on the neural detection of safety, through the polyvagal process of "neuroception," SSP equips therapists with a powerful tool to help their clients become more open and receptive to therapeutic interventions.

This is why many Somatic Experiencing (SE) therapists have seamlessly integrated SSP into their practices. Once understood as a "neural exercise" that promotes greater state regulation and autonomic flexibility, SSP complements the SE concepts of titration (experiencing contraction with minimal autonomic nervous system activation) and pendulation (the innate rhythm between contraction and expansion), which are essential in building resilience.

This is a book that will enrich clinicians' understanding of the fundamental nature of defense and safety, offering practical solutions for creating more effective therapeutic outcomes. It is also a book for anyone seeking a deeper understanding of safety and greater self-compassion.

Peter A. Levine, PhD
author of *In an Unspoken Voice: How the Body Releases Trauma and Restores Goodness* and *An Autobiography of Trauma: A Healing Journey*

Introduction

Retuning the Autonomic Nervous System to Generate Change and Connection

Stefan, a retired submariner, was initially skeptical about the effectiveness of SSP. His wife had suggested it to him, but he doubted that a listening therapy would be any different from listening to the radio. Although he didn't think he needed therapy, he decided to try it, almost to prove his wife wrong. However, much to his surprise, during SSP he noticed that the constant, involuntary bouncing of his leg suddenly stopped. He started sleeping better than he could remember. Surprisingly, his acidic stomach, which he had assumed was normal, also improved. Additionally, he found himself less bad-tempered and argumentative, traits he had always considered just part of who he was. Three years later, these changes have mostly endured.

Safe and Sound Protocol (SSP) is a noninvasive therapy based on Polyvagal Theory (PVT) that involves listening to music that has been filtered to prioritize the frequencies of human speech. This auditory input enables the nervous system to be receptive to cues of safety and to downregulate defensiveness. SSP doesn't rely on your intentions, beliefs, or effort; it works because it engages the nervous system directly without requiring mental or verbal processing.

Feeling safe is a powerful remedy for trauma and dysregulation. Abundant cues of safety are required to offset nervous system imbalance to facilitate connection, change, and healing. This notion is central to SSP and is rooted in PVT.

Polyvagal Theory: The Foundation of Safe and Sound Protocol

Polyvagal Theory (PVT)[1] is the foundational concept behind Safe and Sound Protocol (SSP) and provides insight into why it is so effective. PVT highlights the crucial role of the body and nervous system in health and well-being, demonstrating how our thoughts, emotions, and behaviors are shaped by our body's ongoing assessment of our level of safety or threat. It underscores the bidirectional communication between the body and the brain and the necessity of fostering safety and connection to enhance overall health.

While the origins of PVT are based on neuroanatomy and neurophysiology, its practical application lies in understanding and improving our lived experience. At its core, PVT is a forgiving and hopeful theory about our nervous system, and understanding more about it gives new insights into human behavior. Using a polyvagal lens, we can see the world and how we live in it in a more positive way. A polyvagal approach to life invites curiosity and enhances our experiences and relationships.

PVT elucidates how trauma, illness, disorders, and life experiences can retune the nervous system away from homeostasis and resilience to become trapped in a state of threat and defensiveness, manifested as anxiety, depression, or shutdown. Such defensiveness, while adaptive for survival, constricts our thinking, hinders our ability to connect with others for support, and makes it challenging to feel at ease.

In fact, at the core of many mental, behavioral, and physical health challenges is a nervous system stuck in a state of chronic defense. A medicalized approach to these challenges can sometimes fall short and even pathologize or stigmatize a person by labeling them as unwell. By focusing instead on the intricate connection between the brain and body as PVT does, we hope clinicians will have a more compassionate and understanding perspective toward their clients. Individuals, in turn, can deepen their awareness of themselves—sensations, thoughts, emotions, and behaviors included.

SSP, in line with this approach, aims to rebalance the nervous system to restore optimal health and equanimity. Detailed in chapter 2, this evidence-based protocol has successfully helped hundreds of thousands of people retune their nervous systems and cultivate a stronger sense of safety.

Insight from Diverse Cases

The diverse case stories of SSP in the second part of this book show that when the nervous system regains its capacity to feel safe, individuals can express themselves genuinely, engage comfortably with others, and embrace a life of greater openness and ease. What we all want is to feel safe enough to be who we are, in all of our insights, intelligence, creativity, benevolence, and compassion. SSP serves as a catalyst, guiding individuals toward a state of safety and connection by helping the nervous system restore its fundamental balance and flexibility.

Here are three short vignettes of SSP experiences that illustrate how each client was able to better connect with the people in their life and to live with authenticity and joy.

A Child Moving from Self-Regulation to Co-Regulation

Mateo was a shy, autistic four-year-old who could not sustain eye contact or engage socially due to his unique sensory sensitivities and communication style. He attended regular sessions with Christine, his occupational therapist, to listen to SSP. He was offered an array of toys organized in colored bins to play with while listening to the filtered music of SSP. Mateo chose the same two bins of plastic dinosaurs, cars, and trucks to play with during each SSP session. During the first two SSP sessions, he was laser-focused on lining up the dinosaurs and vehicles by size, color, and type. This was an adaptive strategy he used for self-regulation and comfort during unfamiliar situations.

During the third session, he made the dinosaurs walk around, and he drove the cars and trucks in circles, smiling impishly up at Christine. This was the first time he had ever sought out eye contact with her. In the fourth session, he made a dinosaur drive a truck, giggling at the silliness. His body language was more open, his face lit up with his smile, and he showed a sense of playfulness and curiosity that Christine hadn't seen before. In the last session of SSP, he picked up two cars, handed one to Christine, and started to drive his car, making it clear that she should do the same. Their mutual delight in the back-and-forth play was palpable.

Mateo transitioned from relying on a robust internal locus of control and a preference for routine and predictability to welcoming reciprocal connection, co-regulation, and playfulness. Because of SSP, Mateo was able to build trust with a safe person, a connection that may not otherwise have developed. As a result, his nervous system is now primed for more co-regulatory experiences like this one. His newfound level of connection brought immense joy to his family while also accelerating his progress in motor planning and sensory integration.

A Traumatized Woman Overcomes Lifelong Panic

Years after Teresa's mother fled Germany as a young woman in the 1930s, she suffered from flashbacks of mob violence where she had witnessed multiple murders, including one of a newborn infant, and she herself narrowly escaped death.

When Teresa was eight weeks old, her mother experienced a flashback of those horrors and believed she and Teresa were facing an angry mob. Struggling in a blind frenzy, she unintentionally caused Teresa severe and extensive injuries. This event, its aftermath, and later similar episodes with both parents taught Teresa to avoid others and dissociate when anyone came near. She left home at 18 and soon forgot almost all of her childhood. She created a good life, pursued many interests, but couldn't relax except when alone.

In her midforties, Teresa's senses became increasingly scrambled; she couldn't see and hear at the same time or control her physical movements. She forgot how to dress and tell time. She passed out after eating. Medical doctors could find nothing wrong. Alternative healing methods provided some relief, but, as a side effect, she began having terrifying flashbacks of being hurt by her mother. Upon questioning, her mother confessed and apologized for her violence. Yet Teresa's flashbacks grew worse.

Still seeking help in 2019, Teresa discovered SSP and found that it lifted the crushing weight she'd always carried. She realized that the weight had been a lifelong experience of panic. She completed SSP a second time four months later and became "astonishingly sociable" and able to think in "new, clear-minded ways." Teresa has since completed SSP five more times to peel away additional layers of trauma.

She sees how limited her life was, revels in her new ease especially with self-care, and for the first time, can sense her body and emotions without triggering traumatic replays. Her life is full now: she has many friends she enjoys spending time with, participates in group activities, and even performs comedy.

Digging Out of a Dark Hole of Alienation and Long COVID

Omar was a Muslim teenager in London when the world was shaken by the tragic events of September 11, 2001. After that, like many Muslims, he experienced suspicion, discrimination, and hostility due to his faith.

Over the years, he became deeply involved in political activism, working passionately to fight against government and media discrimination. In June of 2021, he tested positive for COVID and his infection progressed into Long COVID. He experienced breathing difficulties, extreme chronic fatigue, dysregulation, and difficulty sitting up or standing. He searched desperately for remedies and tried various ones with limited success. When he finally connected with an SSP provider, he had been housebound for almost a year and needed to lie down for their virtual sessions.

Omar immediately resonated with the ideas of PVT shared by his SSP provider as it answered so many questions about his own experiences, including his behaviors and those of others in his past. He was able to identify the "siege" mentality he took on in the post-9/11 environment, seeking to protect himself and his community from discrimination, though leaving him in a heightened state of vigilance. During this period, he found the safety and community he craved by joining various Muslim groups. When incriminating information about some of his own religious leaders emerged, the perspective of

PVT allowed him to remain curious, despite the deep spiritual questioning and feelings of rage this triggered.

After months of weekly sessions of slowly titrated SSP, Omar gradually gained new health and energy. He went from using a wheelchair to walking and driving a car again. While previously he had no concentration and was unable even to read a single page of an academic book, he is now pursuing a PhD at Cambridge University. He credits SSP and his provider equally for helping him to "find his way out of a very dark hole." While he still feels somewhat vulnerable, he knows he is on a positive journey of growth and healing.

The unexpected and quite different changes resulting from SSP that Stefan, Mateo, Teresa, and Omar experienced are possible because of how SSP can affect our autonomic nervous system (ANS), which is central to our physical and mental health. SSP can adjust the central control dial of our nervous system to retune it and help to shift it toward balance and ease. As you will learn, this control dial is in the brainstem, the nexus of the body-brain connection. By infusing a sense of safety, SSP initiates feedback loops that can change the settings of the central control dial. This shifts the nervous system away from defensiveness and toward a greater capacity for social connection, the ability to accommodate stressors, and better health.

About Us and Our Vision for This Book

To provide context for how SSP came to be, we will start with a brief introduction to our background and work. Stephen W. Porges is a world-renowned and distinguished neuroscientist, the developer of PVT, and the creator of SSP. He has published more than 500 peer-reviewed papers that have been cited over 60,000 times and six books on PVT. Karen Onderko has been instrumental in bringing SSP from the laboratory to the clinical world, conducting the initial testing, developing the early training, creating delivery guidelines, and supporting the SSP provider community.

We conceived the idea of a book of case studies in 2017 during the early stages of SSP's release and adoption by clinicians. As stories of change and connection flooded in, each offering valuable insights, the potential for a comprehensive exploration was realized. Through the enthusiasm of the early SSP provider community, the breadth of the possibilities and applications of SSP was clear and compelling.

Case studies and stories formed SSP's foundational evidence base upon which clinical trials, randomized controlled trials, and real-world evidence were added. We envisioned a book that utilized cases to illustrate how PVT not only unveils the roots of clinical symptoms but also demonstrates how SSP can alleviate them and enhance overall well-being.

How SSP Came to Be

SSP was developed based on Steve's optimistic belief that the nervous system's flexibility could be adjusted to encourage spontaneous engagement, co-regulation, and trust. Over years of research, he noticed that the state of one's nervous system (their "autonomic state") and their behavior were closely linked. By identifying physiological markers that indicate a tendency to be under- or overreactive, he created a treatment model. This model focuses on changing the autonomic state that predisposes a person to react, rather than addressing the reaction itself. Traditionally, therapeutic strategies aimed to change responses like behavior, thoughts, or physiological reactions to stimuli. His approach shifts this focus to adjusting the autonomic state, which can restore the natural ability for engagement, flexibility, and resilience. For a full vision of how the protocol came to be, we share Steve's personal journey with SSP and the history of its evolution below (a more detailed account can be found on this book's bonus page online: soundstrue.com/safe-and-sound-bonus).

The Prehistory of SSP

Between 1985 and 2001, as a faculty member at the University of Maryland, Steve was interested in the autonomic and behavioral regulation of autistic children. At that time, since he was formulating PVT, he was curious if features of individuals' interactive social behavior were dependent on their autonomic state. Based on his research he hypothesized that poor autonomic regulation was foundational and that signals of calming and safety would be supportive. As PVT evolved, he began to understand the profound signaling power of melodic vocalizations in calming. He started to use the mother's vocal calming of an infant and our vocal engagement of our mammalian pets as a model for a potential intervention.

Creating and Researching an Early Version of SSP

By the late 1990s Steve had spent hundreds of hours observing autistic children. He witnessed the behavioral defensiveness of these children and their hypersensitivities and intuitively wanted to calm their nervous system to enable them to feel more comfortable in their bodies. He envisioned a way that was totally different from the treatment models that emphasized behavioral modification techniques, which were prevalent in the 1990s. Steve wondered if PVT would provide the insights to craft such an intervention. Thus, the initial SSP was prototyped as a stealth intervention that communicated with the hardwired circuits that the calming prosodic vocalizations of a mother's lullaby intuitively recruited. The prototype was called the Listening Project Protocol (LPP).

Steve envisaged a neural exercise in which the acoustic signal (filtered music) would be delivered to the child's nervous system through a narrow frequency band that would be available even when in a defensive state. The frequency band of the music would progressively expand and contract until the child experienced and welcomed the full frequency band of social communication; that is, the acoustic frequencies through which human vocalizations are used for social communication. Steve theorized that as the acoustic frequency band expanded and contracted, the neural regulation of structures involved in social engagement linking the muscles of the face and head with the calming influence of the vagus nerve (see chapter 1) on the heart would become available.

Steve viewed hypersensitivity and gaze aversion as natural responses to perceived threats by the ANS. While common in autistic individuals, these behaviors are seen as adaptive rather than pathological. PVT suggests that sensory issues, central to autism diagnoses, may lessen when the nervous system feels safe, such as through LPP. This nonjudgmental approach respects neurodiversity while promoting calmness to reduce hypersensitivity. LPP and PVT emphasize the importance of foundational states, such as calmness or feeling threatened, which higher brain functions rely on, rather than the higher brain processes typically associated with neurodiversity.

During the initial pilot study, Steve and his research colleagues observed children sharing and exhibiting reciprocal play behaviors. Their most poignant memory of initial reactions to the LPP is that of a child who would not tolerate a headset. They adapted to the challenge by placing speakers in a special sound-attenuated cube built with sound-dampening blankets attached to PVC pipes with Velcro fasteners. Once this hypersensitive nonverbal child entered the cube and heard the computer-altered music, he clearly articulated one word: "Safe."

Documentation began on how the "stealth" intervention profoundly reduced hypersensitivities, improved auditory processing, promoted sharing behaviors, improved emotional control, and enhanced spontaneous social engagement. Laboratory assessments were paralleled by parent and teacher reports reflecting calmer, happier, and more interactive children.

Transitioning from LPP to SSP

In January 2016, Steve was approached by Integrated Listening Systems (iLs), an acoustic therapy company. The interests of iLs were aligned with the goals for LPP, and iLs already had an extensive customer base of pediatric occupational therapists, physical therapists (PTs), and speech therapists. These factors led to an agreement to pursue distribution of the LPP. A group of occupational therapists (OTs) and speech therapists beta-tested the LPP for three months. The findings from the group were very positive, with excellent reports of efficacy and zero concerns about safety.

The name of the therapy was changed by the authors of this book to the Safe and Sound Protocol. The name was crafted to honor the important role that feeling safe (i.e., being in a ventral vagal state) played in mediating the accessibility of the client's nervous system to the sound.

It acknowledged that being in an autonomic state that supported feelings of safety was obligatory for the nervous system to benefit from the acoustic exposure.

SSP was released as a therapy to the clinical world quietly in March of 2017. The protocol for delivery of SSP was the same as that used in the two foundational studies on SSP with children where it had shown to be safe and effective: one hour of listening for five consecutive days.[2]

In mid-2019, Unyte Health, a provider of nervous system solutions that support awareness, regulation, and resilience, purchased iLs and immediately began creating a mobile application to access and listen to SSP. It was being tested and rolled out just as the COVID pandemic was beginning. Unyte Health continues to expand the user base, enhance training, update SSP playlists, and offer support for providers by developing best practice guidelines.

The Evolution of SSP

The clinicians who were the early adopters of SSP came in two waves. First were the pediatric therapists such as OTs, PTs, speech therapists, child psychologists, and educators who supported children with neurodevelopmental disorders, early life traumas, autism spectrum disorder, and genetic disorders such as Down syndrome and Fragile X syndrome. In the second wave were psychologists, psychotherapists, social workers, and body-based therapists who worked with adults with developmental trauma, post-traumatic stress disorder (PTSD), complex trauma, attention deficit hyperactivity disorder (ADHD), addiction, chronic pain, anxiety, and depression.

The early responses were astonishing. New stories of change were reported almost daily. Clinicians were so moved by their clients' responses to SSP that they formed communities to study PVT, share stories, debate best delivery practices, and support each other. One parent started an SSP Facebook group for parents when her son was set on a new trajectory after receiving SSP. PVT book groups, Facebook groups for clinicians, and SSP study groups emerged organically.

The therapy was working especially well for younger clients. Some children were becoming more verbal, and behavioral reactivity was reduced once more resilience was introduced to their nervous system. There were very few negative reactions; those that did occur were related to a "two steps forward, one step back" effect in development. Examples of these temporary regressions included bedwetting, clinginess, and baby talk, but they typically resolved quickly.

Providers were enthusiastic about the results they were seeing, and SSP grew by word of mouth. Some clinicians described how glad they were that they didn't retire before SSP was released. Others began taking new clients only if they were willing to do SSP since it made the work with their other modalities so much more effective.

Being Guided by Providers

As the number of providers grew, so did the number of disciplines represented. But in time, mental health professionals working with adults who experienced anxiety, depression, and the effects of trauma began noticing different responses. For some clients, SSP evoked vulnerabilities they were not yet ready to address. Some clients felt discomfort and wanted to stop the music. Other clients who may have had very little access to their bodily senses or interoception may not have been aware that they were experiencing a shift into a defensive state and were unable to give accurate feedback of their potential dysregulation.

The most common problem was that some clients experienced the cues of safety in the filtered music as cues of threat. Many traumas stem from interpersonal abuse perpetrated by individuals in a caretaking and trusted position. Signals of safety subconsciously became inseparable from feelings of threat for those with such experiences. The distilled essence of safety embedded in the music drew their physiology to lower its defenses. But this subconscious vulnerability was intolerable, triggering defensive states within their nervous systems and causing distress and dysregulation.

The SSP provider community, driven by a shared desire to exchange insights and comprehend their observations, offered examples of how these defensive reactions manifested. They met in groups online and shared ideas on social media of how to respond to them. It was clear that the reported adverse responses were related to the ANS.

Adjusting the Protocol

Initially, Steve was distraught over the possibility that SSP could be destabilizing to some. He had designed SSP based on the premise that our nervous system literally had no choice but to reflexively, via a neuroception of safety, become accessible when exposed to the modulation of acoustic frequencies within the frequency band of social communication. He wondered if there was a flaw in his reasoning. He was so concerned that he wanted to limit the use of SSP to avoid the potential of triggering defensive reactions.

The SSP provider community convinced Steve that they would figure out how to harness the power of SSP for individuals with adversity histories. The providers realized that the signals embedded in SSP were powerful, and their client's bodily reactions needed to be respected. This led to adjusting the protocol to allow a slower delivery to provide the client's nervous system sufficient time to resolve the disruption. For some clients, the disruption recovered almost immediately. But for others it took a few hours or even days. Insightful therapists closely monitored their clients' reactions and titrated the delivery of SSP to match the accessibility of the client's nervous system. With this new insight into how SSP could be used, trauma-informed therapists observed accelerated improvements of the clients as they intertwined SSP with other trauma-informed therapies.

Pragmatically, outcomes improved from slowing delivery and matching delivery with the client's autonomic state, which could be monitored by listening to the client's voice, looking at the client's facial expressions, gesture, and posture, and asking the client about their bodily feelings.

Trauma-informed therapists could use SSP to support their clients in expanding their capacity to accept and process signals leading to accessibility. They could also gain a better appreciation of the powerful adaptive reactions that their nervous system employs to protect them.

Even in those with adverse reactions, SSP was doing what it was designed to do. This knowledge gave reassurance and confidence to providers that SSP was a potent tool with tremendous possibility when delivered carefully.

Less Is More and Other Early Learnings

The goal of going slowly is not only to avoid overstimulation or shutdown but also to access the full benefits of the SSP delivery process. More signals of safety do not make one safer. Instead, they can lead to hypersensitivities, emotional volatility, and even shutdown. "Less is more" became a mantra of SSP delivery. By going slowly, the provider and client can take the time that is needed to process and integrate how the body is taking in these signals. Each step can be savored.

Since each person's ANS is unique, every SSP delivery will have its own pace. And each session will be different. What the client has experienced in their life in the intervening days or weeks will have had an effect on them. And the same is true of the provider. Each session is another experience of getting to know each other, and an opportunity to get to know each other's nervous systems.

Best Practices

Best practices for delivering SSP continue to evolve due to the thoughtfulness and brilliance of the SSP provider community. The early learnings and mantras of "Less is more" and "Safe before sound" hold true as new ideas and applications continue to be shared. With the goal to optimize its effectiveness and minimize potential discomfort or hyperstimulation, a set of precautions was created.

The Foundational SSP Training is constantly evolving, and SSP providers are increasingly sharing their individual approaches through mentoring, clinical consultations, Q&As, and webinars. Additionally, specific guidelines on using SSP together with another modality (for example, eye movement desensitization and reprocessing [EMDR], Somatic Experiencing, and occupational therapy) continue to be created by practitioners who specialize in both SSP and their specific modality.

Continuous Learning

While SSP is an easy tool to use, it requires an attuned presence and nuanced approach to deliver it safely and effectively. It presents a new way of working with people that takes time, experience, and compassion to refine. There will always be a learning curve to working with SSP because each person—along with their nervous system—is unique.

SSP is ultimately a hopeful tool that is rewarding to both the provider and the client. Providers have found it a privilege to work at the level of the nervous system and a joy to witness how adopting the lens of PVT can change a person's outlook and soften their view of themselves and the world.

In the real case studies presented in part 2 of this book, you will see the potential in people that SSP reveals. You will also see that when one person improves their nervous system regulation and vagal tone, it can create ripples of connection and openheartedness within a relationship, family, workplace, and community.

As a scientist, Steve is thrilled that PVT has led to a helpful intervention. It was the commitment, curiosity, and compassion of the SSP provider community in collaboration with their clients that was fundamental to the tremendous evolution of SSP delivery. This collaboration continues to be encouraged. The ongoing evolution of SSP promises growth and possibilities. Steve continues to listen and learn from client and provider experiences.

About This Book

Consider this book a welcome mat to understanding the potential for healing and transforming the body and brain by working with the ANS, particularly using SSP. It is written for both clinicians and laypeople who are curious to know more about their health and how to improve it. You will find insights into PVT, the adaptive mechanisms of the ANS, and especially how practical methods, SSP in particular, can relieve chronic defensiveness and give hope.

Part 1

Part 1 of the book provides an overview of the science behind the ANS, PVT, and SSP. Each chapter provides ample theory, practice, tools, and approaches to consider and adopt. Throughout part 1, you will learn about your innate capacity for health, growth, and restoration. You'll discover the centrality of the nervous system to physical and mental health. By understanding PVT, the foundation of SSP, you may gain a deeper awareness of the autonomic states your own nervous system traverses. With this knowledge, you can become more attuned to these patterns and how they impact your life.

The first three chapters in part 1 focus on the science of the nervous system, PVT, and SSP while the fourth chapter provides practices for working with your nervous system:

- Chapter 1 describes how our physiological state is the intervening variable between stimulus and response and that an understanding of our capacity to respond rather than react can be cultivated.

- Chapter 2 focuses on SSP, describing what it is and how it is different from most other therapies. It also reviews SSP's clinical research and real-world evidence base.

- Chapter 3 investigates SSP's capacity to effect change, how it was developed based on PVT, the way in which it works, and why it is so often used to support other therapeutic modalities.

- Chapter 4 contains the Regulation Toolbox, which offers personalized activities to support your nervous system.

The neuroscience in part 1 is intended to develop a deeper understanding of how PVT and SSP work. Lay readers are welcome to peruse these more technical passages, but it's not necessary to fully engage with all the science to understand how SSP works and why it's effective. If you have less interest in the content in part 1, feel free to begin with the case stories in part 2, which offer insights into the important role SSP can play in the brain-body connection. Once you've experienced the possibilities of a nervous system approach, you may want to come back to the science for a deeper exploration.

Part 2

Part 2 of the book presents real-world case studies of SSP and showcases the art behind the science of PVT in how providers deliver SSP. The cases illustrate SSP's effectiveness in addressing issues such as anxiety, depression, chronic pain, grief, dissociation, and addiction. In each case, we share the client's story, their history and concerns, how SSP was delivered by the provider, and what results emerged. We further discuss and deconstruct each case through the lens of PVT. Each case begins with an overview. You can read the cases in the order they are presented or use the overviews to select cases that align with your interests and concerns or those of your clients.

SSP, delivered by a supportive, co-regulating provider, is an immersive sensory experience that cannot be taught or experienced in a book. The cases portray, again and again, how shifting away from a survival physiology toward one of connection and regulation can unlock previously unseen potential and opportunities. These inspiring accounts show that we can leverage our own neurobiology to reverse downward spirals, cultivate greater resilience and connection, and enjoy a fuller life.

A Word about Safety

The concept of safety is foundational to PVT. However, while PVT is objective, the experience of safety is subjective. What feels "safe" is unique to each person and each situation they face. There is no definition that can describe safety in a way that will resonate with every person because safety is relative. It is shaped by individual experiences, past and present, and the surrounding environment. It is a felt sense[3] that fosters an openness to trust and connection with others.

Due to its integral role in PVT, the word *safe* is used throughout this book. However, if you or a loved one do not experience foundational security, or if the term *safe* is a trigger or causes discomfort, consider using *safe enough* or *enough trust* when you read the words *safe* or *safety* in these pages.

Support and Inclusivity: Navigating the Content and Principles of This Book

Due to its content, it's possible that some of the science in part 1 and the case stories in part 2 may provoke discomfort or distress. Pace your reading and reach out for support if needed as you absorb these stories and concepts. We encourage readers to prioritize self-care throughout their engagement with this book and, with that in mind, we offer the nervous system regulation practices provided in chapter 4.

The aim of this book is to be inclusive of the experiences of all readers, yet we're aware that we cannot understand or address all diverse perspectives and experiences. Whatever your personal experience is, it is valid and unique to you. The principles and techniques outlined in this book are universal because they address fundamental aspects of human nature. SSP engages the nervous system regardless of individual differences and life experiences. Similarly, PVT addresses the wide continuum of psychological and physiological states without judgment. The principles and ideas of this work are about allowing you to become the person you were meant to be and to reach your full potential.

By writing about PVT and SSP, we aim to demonstrate that it's not only possible to suffer less but also to foster more meaningful and fulfilling connections. We hope to show that SSP can be a lifelong gift, empowering individuals to understand their unique nervous systems and develop tools for a calmer, more resilient life. As people's experiences improve, the positive effects ripple out, impacting their entire community. We hope this book will spark curiosity and inspire you to discover how PVT and SSP can benefit not just you but also your friends, family, and clients.

The Autonomic Nervous System, Polyvagal Theory, and Safe and Sound Protocol

Part One

art 1 delves into the transformative power of the autonomic nervous system (ANS), polyvagal theory (PVT), and Safe and Sound Protocol (SSP). Their synergistic relationship can strengthen the brain, body, nervous system, and relationships.

Understanding Behavior and the Nervous System Through PVT

Contrary to the common belief that our behavior is entirely intentional, much of it is actually governed by the state of our nervous system. PVT explains this by showing how our sensations, thoughts, and emotions are deeply influenced by the ANS. This perspective is both forgiving and hopeful. By exploring the science of feeling safe, as PVT is sometimes called, you'll gain a deeper understanding of your ANS and learn how to navigate life with greater ease and connection.

The Role of SSP

As a polyvagal approach, SSP harnesses the power of the ANS to help people live authentically and foster deep, meaningful connections with others. This science-based, natural method leverages the body's intrinsic link between the ANS and well-being to enhance both mental and physical health.

Chapter 1

The Autonomic Nervous System Through the Lens of Polyvagal Theory

The state of our ANS significantly shapes our health and overall well-being. A balanced ANS plays a crucial role in maintaining homeostasis across essential physiological functions and fostering optimal conditions for the body's natural healing processes. Moreover, it supports emotional resilience, mental clarity, and meaningful connections with others. In contrast, dysregulation of the ANS can lead to a spectrum of disruptions, including anxiety, depression, sleep disturbances, fatigue, and chronic pain.

Familiarity with the ANS provides a vital context for comprehending PVT and SSP, both of which can facilitate healing, resilience, connection, and overall well-being. PVT offers insights into how our nervous system reacts to stress and threat, and how we can transition to a state of safety and connection. SSP helps regulate the ANS by utilizing auditory stimulation to promote safety and calmness.

The architecture of the ANS is remarkably intricate and far-reaching, extending its influence across much of the body. This vast network of nerve fibers extends from the brain and spinal cord to organs and tissue throughout the body, terminating in the abdomen. Like carbon fiber, which is both strong and lightweight, it provides a robust and flexible foundation for our physical and emotional health.

The ANS

The ANS is the division of the peripheral nervous system that governs involuntary bodily functions. It controls our heart rate, blood pressure, breathing, digestion, metabolism, bladder function, body temperature, reproductive processes, and internal organ functions. It also profoundly influences our sensations, thoughts, emotions, and behaviors. Fundamentally, the ANS plays an essential role in keeping the body and brain dynamically operating in an optimal and balanced range to adapt to the ever-changing demands of our environment.

The ANS functions as a bidirectional communication network connecting our bodily organs with our brain. Although we tend to think that the cerebral cortex of the brain is the primary regulator of the body, we need to reexamine this relationship. When we delve deeper into this bidirectionality, we recognize the profound influence that our bodily organs have on our ability to think, feel good, accurately interpret signals in our environment, and connect with others. Once we grasp this relationship, we become more aware of the dynamic interplay between the feelings of our body and the mental activity we use to frame experience. Not only are we aware that thoughts may shift our physiological state, but now we understand that our physiological state actively plays a role in limiting or expanding the range of our experiences by biasing our perspective from being defensive to being curious, engaging, playful, and explorative.

Because it manages our bodily functions and emotional states without our conscious control, the ANS is commonly referred to as the "automatic" nervous system. However, we can influence our ANS to support its functioning and positively impact our health and well-being. Nervous system regulation practices, such as breathing exercises, therapy, sociality, and SSP can support a flexible and balanced ANS.

When the ANS becomes dysregulated, it can disrupt both acute and long-term systemic processes, impacting our physical and mental health. The nervous system is designed to respond to threats and revert to an internal balance once the alarming event subsides. Nonhuman mammals typically experience an immediate and complete stress response: levels of stress hormones like cortisol and adrenaline surge, activating the body to confront the danger. But once the threat dissipates, many animals literally "shake it off."

In contrast, modern humans often experience an incomplete or prolonged stress response. We might react to perceived threats and then become stuck in a state of activation or shutdown. This can make us less inclined to use movement to discharge residual tension, leading to rumination on past stressors.

For instance, if you are worried you may be laid off from your job, you might spiral into self-doubt, replaying work interactions in your mind and analyzing your performance. Your heart rate and blood pressure might increase, your breathing could become shallow, and your muscles could tense as levels of stress hormones like cortisol surge. All of this could happen in the relative safety of your own living room.

When our threat response extends into long-term chronic defensiveness and hypervigilance, our systems become fatigued. While stress hormones are crucial in acute situations, prolonged high levels can have a negative effect on various bodily systems, resulting in chronic inflammation, sleep problems, brain fog, poor digestion, blood sugar imbalance, or other adverse effects. Sustained vigilance and stress become metabolically costly, steadily eroding both physical and mental health. Our bodily systems require time for health, growth, and restoration, but chronic defensiveness impedes this natural healing capability.

Dysregulation of the ANS can have both short-term and long-term effects on our physical and mental health. Short-term dysregulation may manifest as elevated heart rate and blood pressure, rapid breathing, and heightened alertness. If dysregulation persists, such as in complex trauma, it can induce chronic stress that impacts the immune system, inflammation, cardiovascular health, and overall well-being. Emotionally, short-term dysregulation may cause reactivity and irritability. Long-term emotional dysregulation is associated with mental health disorders such as anxiety, depression, sleep disturbances, and cognitive impairment. A chart detailing the effects of ANS dysregulation on our physical and mental health can be found in appendix 2.

While the ANS can be disrupted in many ways, it can also act as a ballast, providing stability as we navigate the complexities of life. With a balanced nervous system, we can recover more quickly from stressors, regulate our emotional health, and meet challenges with greater equanimity. We are available for social engagement, empathy, and co-regulation. Physiologically, we have better heart and digestive health, immune function, and sleep quality, clearer thinking, and improved memory and problem-solving skills. The body can heal more easily when the nervous system is balanced and not locked in states of threat.

PVT as a Neural Navigator

PVT provides a forgiving and hopeful explanation of how our nervous system evolved to be inextricably linked to our physical and mental health.

The primary role of our brain and body is to keep us alive. Because of this, we have processes that operate continuously outside of our conscious awareness to scan the environment for signs of danger and safety. These signals are swiftly processed through the nervous system and we react, before we even understand why, with shifts in our autonomic—or physiological—state.

Often referred to as "the science of feeling safe," PVT[1] explains how our body's appraisal of safety affects our sensations, thoughts, emotions, and behaviors. To fully engage in the world, we need to feel safe, but safety is not merely the absence of danger or threat. Safety involves a feeling of ease in the moment that promotes sociality, adaptability, and co-regulation with another. Co-regulation describes a harmonious relationship that enriches each person's sense of self, enabling reciprocal nervous system regulation that promotes balance and well-being.

When we experience symptoms of mental or physical distress, it often means our nervous system is not sensing enough safety and has shifted into a defensive state. This defensiveness limits access to healthy social connections, clear thinking, openness to new ideas and perspectives, and the potential for health, growth, and restoration. For example, during a high-stakes presentation, nervousness can hinder clear communication, lead to forgetfulness, and inhibit the ability to build rapport with the audience. The greater the threat, the more serious the consequences.

Historically, the ANS was considered an antagonistic two-branch system. One was either in a parasympathetic ("rest and digest") or a sympathetic ("fight or flight") state. The parasympathetic branch supports our ability to rest when needed, socialize when desired, and heal, grow, and learn in ways that support the normal functions of the body to keep us healthy. The sympathetic branch helps activate us for work, exercise, and play and also triggers the well-known fight-or-flight response when facing a threat. It prepares our body for defense, whether through actual fighting, fleeing or, more commonly, engaging in aggressive, hypervigilant, or avoidant behaviors.

In contrast to this binary system, PVT describes a more nuanced, three-part system of physiological states resulting from real or perceived sensations of threat or safety. The term *polyvagal* (*poly* implying "more than one" and *vagal* referring to the vagus nerve) was chosen to underscore how the theory further divides the parasympathetic branch of the ANS into two additional subbranches—ventral and dorsal—to reflect two pathways of the vagus nerve.

The Vagus Nerve

The vagus nerve, the 10th of 12 pairs of cranial nerves, is a crucial component of the ANS. It carries extensive bidirectional information between the brain and the body, more than any other cranial nerve. Cranial nerves, distinct from the spinal nerves, emerge directly from the brain to control sensory and motor functions in the head and neck including sight, smell, hearing, taste, movement, and vocalization. They transmit sensory information from specific organs to the brainstem (via afferent pathways) as well as motor commands from the brainstem back to these organs (via efferent pathways).

Among the cranial nerves, the vagus nerve is unique in extending beyond the head and neck. It is the longest cranial nerve, running from the brainstem down to the abdomen where it connects with all the internal organs. Along this extensive pathway, the vagus nerve, in conjunction with other cranial nerves, influences various physiological functions, including facial expressions, hearing, vocal tone, heart rate, breathing patterns, posture, and the function of visceral organs. Contrary to the notion that the brain governs the body, 80 to 90 percent of the information transmitted through the vagus nerve travels from the body to the brain.

The vagus nerve is actually a pair of nerves, one on each side of the body, and it has two components: ventral and dorsal. These terms refer to their origins in the brainstem—*ventral* (front) and *dorsal* (back). Both components belong to the parasympathetic nervous system but serve different functions.

The ventral vagal pathway is myelinated, meaning its neuronal connections have a protective fatty coating called myelin, allowing for faster transmission of nerve signals. It regulates organs located above the diaphragm. The ventral vagus originates in the nucleus ambiguus, an area of the brainstem linked to the neural regulation of the muscles of our face and head, which are essential for social engagement. The ventral vagus integrates the regulation of blood pressure and heart rate with vocalizations, hearing acuity, posture, and facial expressions—all critical for fostering social interactions, cooperation, and trust. It acts like a "vagal brake" on the heart, slowing heart rate when engaged and increasing it when released.

The dorsal vagal pathway is evolutionarily ancient and unmyelinated, regulating organs below the diaphragm. Originating from an area of the brainstem called the dorsal motor nucleus, the dorsal vagus is an important neural regulator of the stomach, digestive tract, and other organs. In a state of safety, it fosters digestion and supports calm, safe bonding behaviors, such as nursing a baby. In response to danger, it's linked to fainting, fear-induced defecating, shutting down, and dissociating in response to overwhelming threats.

Constructs Describing Vagal Function
The following constructs have been used to describe how the vagus functionally supports autonomic state, bodily processes, and social engagement.

Heart Rate Variability

Heart rate variability (HRV) reflects neural regulation of the heart. It is measured by the variation in the time between heartbeats. A healthy heart does not beat with a constant rate—only a heart without nervous system control would beat at a relatively constant rate. For example, as we exhale, the calming influence of the parasympathetic nervous system, via the vagus, is engaged, leading to a decrease in our heart rate. When we inhale, the vagal influence is depressed, enabling sympathetic influences to functionally increase our heart rate. The greater the variation in the time between heartbeats, the higher HRV will be. In general, vagal pathways provide the prominent neural influence contributing to HRV. Higher HRV typically correlates with better health, reflects a nervous system that is flexible and capable of adapting fluidly to changing demands, and is thus associated with health, growth, and healing. Lower HRV can signal stress, fatigue, or underlying health issues.

Vagal Tone and Respiratory Sinus Arrhythmia

Vagal tone, or more accurately "ventral" vagal tone, reflects the activity of the ventral vagus nerve, specifically, how well the vagus nerve can slow heart rate to promote relaxation and recovery. Ventral vagal tone produces a respiratory pattern in the beat-to-beat heart rate known as respiratory sinus arrhythmia (RSA). RSA is a component of HRV and a more precise index of cardiac vagal tone than HRV. RSA tends to covary with HRV, and higher values are associated with better access to ease and connection.

Vagal Brake

The vagal brake is the mechanism by which the ventral vagus regulates heart rate. When we feel safe and the ventral vagus is activated, the vagal brake engages and slows our heart rate. Conversely, the vagal brake is released when threat or danger is perceived, causing our heart rate to increase. Engaging and releasing the vagal brake respectively increases and decreases our access to the calmer and more connected ventral vagal state. The vagal brake is fluctuating throughout the day to meet the demands of the situations we encounter.

Vagal Efficiency

Vagal efficiency (VE) is a measure of the robustness of the vagal brake. It is quantified by calculating the relationship between cardiac vagal tone (measured by RSA) and heart rate. Higher VE is associated with more efficient vagal regulation of heart rate and better calming after activities such as exercise and posture shifts, and it reflects one's ability to respond effectively to stressors and maintain homeostasis. Regulating activities, like those described in chapter 4, exercise the vagal brake and can lead to higher vagal tone, HRV, and VE.

Neuroception: Our Subconscious Surveillance System

Neuroception, a term unique to PVT, is a full-body risk detection system that works without our conscious control or awareness. Our neuroception is continuously surveilling our body, our environment, and the experiences we have with other people to detect signals of threat or safety. This information, frequently derived from changes as subtle as a transitory shift in the facial expression of another person, is rapidly relayed between the body and the brain and determines how we react by reflexively altering our autonomic state.

When we detect signals of safety (such as a friend's familiar smile), our vagal brake slows our heart and activates the parasympathetic system allowing for connection. When we detect a threat (like an intimidating tone of voice or a loss of eye contact), the vagal brake releases, our heart rate increases, our breathing becomes more rapid and shallow, and we notice the urge to back away. These cues of safety or threat are not processed cognitively. We respond to them without thinking until we notice a change in our body like being drawn toward or deterred by an experience.

Just as our neuroception is always monitoring our own experience, so is the neuroception of others monitoring us. A sense of security in the world is not only detected *by* us but *of* us as well. Our nervous system is both receiving *and* sending information about our surroundings. Beneath our awareness, we are in constant interaction with our environment and the people in it.

Neuroception both influences and is influenced by our current autonomic state. Naturally biased toward the negative, neuroception may err on the side of caution to increase our chance of survival. A defensive state can cause us to be overly vigilant to our environment, and we may respond to threats that aren't even there.

When trauma is a factor, the sensitivity of neuroception is recalibrated to a much lower threshold. This may result in situations being interpreted as more dangerous than they actually are. Paradoxically, it can also skew neuroception such that actual physical threats are overlooked or underestimated.

Interoception

Neuroception and interoception are partner systems in the process of detecting safety and risk. Interoception is a sensory system that enables us to feel our internal organs, bodily sensations, and overall condition. It allows for conscious awareness of how cues of safety and threat, via neuroception, impact our body. While neuroception occurs outside of conscious awareness, interoception gives us greater awareness of our autonomic state in the moment.

The insula, a region in the cerebral cortex, plays a central role in interoception, emotional processing, and maintaining balance of the ANS. Receptors in our skin, muscles, and internal organs relay sensory information through the brainstem to the insula, which translates these signals for conscious perception. Sensory information is integrated with emotional and cognitive signals to provide a sense of ourselves in the world. Not only does the insula convey information, but it plays important roles in cognition and motivation, allowing us to make judgments, anticipate consequences, and adjust our behavior.

Practically, when our interoception detects a physical sensation like thirst or cold, we are motivated to drink water or put on a sweater. Likewise, physical sensations, such as an elevated heart rate and "butterflies" in the stomach, alert us to feeling nervous and motivate us to take deep breaths and move to release the tension.

Good interoceptive awareness leads to a better understanding of distinct emotions. When you can finely sense how the feeling of one emotion is different from another and differentiate the intensity of each, you can improve your emotional awareness and gain better control of your emotions.[2]

Autonomic/Physiological State

The nervous system has different modes—or states—that result from our neuroception of safety or threat. Our autonomic state, the current physiological condition of the ANS, influences our sensations, thoughts, emotions, and behavior. It biases our perception of the environment and prepares our physiology to be welcoming or defensive toward people and situations. Different from traits, which are more stable, our states dynamically shift throughout the day to meet our various experiences. Every state serves an adaptive function, crucial for survival in transient situations. However, prolonged or chronic immersion in a defensive state compromises the ANS's capacity to maintain homeostasis and essential functions like health, growth, and restoration. PVT posits a broadened view of the ANS, emphasizing its integration with other physiological processes including endocrine, immune, and neuropeptide. Thus, the terms *autonomic state* and *physiologic state* are used interchangeably in this book.

The Primary States of the ANS

There are three primary autonomic states that functionally promote experiences of being connected, activated, and shutdown. Each has its own quality, behavioral responses, and effects on our physiology and can be further understood with a metaphor, a general description, and a color.

Connected Ventral Vagal State (We Feel Safe)

The connected ventral vagal state is part of the parasympathetic system and is one of safety and social connection. In it, we feel safe. We're accessible and can engage authentically and collaboratively with others. We can be compassionate, creative, and engage in life with ease. We are available for health, growth, and restoration.

Our heart rate and blood pressure are steady, our breathing is steady, and oxytocin is released. Our bodily systems function smoothly, and we have full access to our cognition.

- Metaphor: We are floating in an inflatable lifeboat—buoyant, easy to maneuver, and able to remain stable despite the wind and waves.

- Description: We might say, "We are floating."

- Color: Green, which is often linked to nature and symbolizes growth, renewal, and vitality.

Activated Sympathetic State (We Feel Threatened and Ready for Fight or Flight)

When we no longer feel safe, and the social strategies of our connected state are not sufficient to address a current situation, the sympathetic state of activation coordinates our mobilization response. This state gives us energy and prepares us for fight or flight. In this defensive state, we are on high alert, aggressive even, and unable to truly connect with others. We may be biased toward perceiving threats where there aren't any.

We feel tense or anxious and lose access to our impulse control, higher cognition, and other executive functions. Our heart rate is elevated and our breathing is rapid and shallow. Cortisol floods our system. Blood flows to our muscles and our strength is increased, our reflexes are faster, and our vision widens while the capacity of bodily functions unnecessary for physical defense, such as digestion, healing, and socialization, decreases.

- Metaphor: We are tipped out of the lifeboat and actively struggling against the waves and currents.

- Description: We might say, "We are flipping out."

- Color: Red, reflecting its function to enhance the flow of blood throughout the body. Interestingly, red is a common signal of danger or warning used in fire alarms, traffic lights, and caution signs.

Shutdown Dorsal Vagal State (We Feel We Are Under an Inescapable Threat and Are Overwhelmed)

When a threat is overwhelming or inescapable, or we are ill or incapacitated, we are shut down and numb. Part of the parasympathetic system, this state is one of disconnection and collapse. Functionally, the shutdown state conserves our metabolic resources. Behaviorally, we may withdraw or collapse in a last-ditch attempt at survival—similar to an animal feigning death. In this state, we feel hopeless, avoidant, and inactive and will sometimes dissociate.

In the shutdown state, we enter a defensive mode leading to physiological changes including the release of natural opioids (endorphins). Blood pressure drops, and heart rate and breathing slow down. Organs below the diaphragm become less active to reduce metabolic demand on the body, which can lead to a sudden evacuation of the bowels. Brain function decreases, resulting in reduced body awareness, impaired cognition, and diminished memory. Threat perception (neuroception) dulls, and we become less aware of our surroundings.

- Metaphor: We sink under the waves to seek protection and avoid the turbulence of the water's surface.

- Description: We might say, "We are flopping down."

- Color: Gray, which can be ominous when associated with the weather and suggests a lack of vitality.

The Natural Sequence of ANS States

The arrangement of autonomic states has historically been referred to as a "hierarchy," which can imply vertical tiers of importance or status. Our states should neither be glorified nor vilified as each state is the appropriate physiological response to our current circumstances. We'll refer here to the natural sequence of states as a "continuum" with movement in both directions.

The three primary physiological states operate in a specific and predictable order. When our neuroception detects safety, we experience the connected, ventral vagal state. This state serves as our home base, offering us the most options for responses and behaviors. When a potential threat becomes apparent, the nervous system initially responds with social engagement and cooperation in an attempt to allay it. If the threat persists, increases, or is sudden, the sympathetic (fight or flight) response is engaged. In cases of overwhelming threat, we move to a dorsal state, leading to shutdown and immobilization. When the threat recedes and cues of safety can once again be detected via neuroception, the system moves back through these states in reverse order, from dorsal through sympathetic to arrive again in a ventral vagal state.

The vagal brake facilitates movement through the continuum of autonomic states. The brake is released for more activation and an increase in heart rate. When the brake is reapplied, the heart slows, and the nervous system moves toward a connected ventral vagal state.

Because of the nuance of the vagal brake, often two or more states can be concurrently active, creating "blended" or "hybrid" states. The primary physiological states are part of a continuum of combined states rather than distinct experiences.

The Continuum of States

The following describes the sequence of how these primary and blended states may present.

Connected (We Feel Safe): Ventral Vagal Pathway

In the connected ventral vagal state, we feel safe and social. We are able to connect and co-regulate with others and have optimal physical functioning and emotional regulation.

Play and Movement (We Feel Safe and Active): Ventral + Sympathetic

Here, our sense of safety allows for an infusion of some activation and mobilization from the sympathetic system. This activation does not involve fear or defensiveness since it is coupled with the ventral vagal pathway of sociality and connection. In this blended state, we are productive and playful and can achieve flow and peak performance levels in many domains.

Quiet Connection and Intimacy (We Feel Safe, Still, and Calm): Ventral + Dorsal

In this blended state, we can be content to be alone or feel the safe presence of another, and we can share moments of intimacy. Defensiveness gives way to safety. Think of a parent cradling their baby whose needs have all been met. This state also allows for moments of intimacy, hugs between close friends, and moments of awe and wonder in nature.

Activated (We Feel Threatened and Ready to Fight or Flee): Sympathetic Nervous System

An activated state prepares us to fight or to flee to escape threat or danger. Threat is not only physical. An activated state can be caused by situations such as financial worries, verbal attacks, bullying, sensory overload, and unexpected or unfamiliar situations. These may lead to physiological responses associated with anxiety, perseverative thinking, and hypervigilance.

Appeasement (Our Threat Signals a Drive to Connect When Options Are Limited): Ventral + Sympathetic + Dorsal

Physiologically, appeasement is the name given to an unconscious mechanism for self-preservation against real or perceived extreme threats. It involves a combination of sympathetic and dorsal defensiveness with oversight by the ventral vagal system. Different from fawning, it uses the social engagement system (SES) to establish rapport and co-regulate the perpetrator or source of the threat.

Appeasement has been described as an "unconscious superpower"—an extreme response in the face of an extreme threat. Many survivors who engaged in appeasing behavior were not aware until after the event that their survival was at risk. Some survivors reported relief and welcome clarity at finding an explanation for the confusing behavior of engaging positively with a person or situation that clearly could have harmed them.[3]

Freeze (We Are Immobilized with Fear): Sympathetic + Dorsal

Like a deer in headlights, sometimes we are paralyzed by fear when we experience a threat that cannot be fought or fled from. In this state, both sympathetic activation and dorsal vagal shutdown are involved. Sympathetic activation is needed to maintain an upright posture and enable an appearance of stillness to avoid detection—perhaps with only our eyes moving. The dorsal vagal state slows our heart rate and breathing to contain our frozen, hiding body.

Shutdown (We Feel We Are Under a Threat We Cannot Escape from and Are Overwhelmed): Dorsal Vagal Pathway

Extreme and overwhelming threats trigger the shutdown dorsal vagal state. Heart rate and breathing slow, and we experience disconnection, dissociation, or numbness.

Fawn (We Submit to Avoid Conflict): Sympathetic + Dorsal

Fawning is a survival response and a means to avoid conflict. It can be embedded in cultural norms or present when power differentials exist. It is compromise with the flavor of submission or compliance.

Fawning involves disarming a perpetrator or power holder so that the individual is seen as subservient and not a threat. Many object to the use of the term *fawn* because it undermines their integrity. Some have proposed *placate* as an alternate descriptor. To placate someone (or a situation) is to make them (it) less hostile by soothing or making concessions. *Placate* may offer a less shameful perspective.

Cyclic Defense Loop (We Are Trapped in a Cycle of Activation and Shutdown): Sympathetic + Dorsal

The cyclic defense loop is characterized by being trapped in an oscillation between the two primary defensive states without access to the ventral vagus and its calming and co-regulatory attributes. Defensive reactions are triggered repeatedly, leading to a cycle of heightened arousal or shutdown.

The perpetuation of the cycle is fueled by how metabolically costly it is to sustain each state. When the energy to remain in a sympathetic state is exhausted, the nervous system shifts to a shutdown dorsal state. Dorsal too, is unsustainable, and a sympathetic state will eventually take over again.

The downward pull of this cyclic repetition can feel relentless and requires potent signals of safety to escape it. People with complex trauma are often trapped in this chronic cycle, which can have devastating effects on relationships and cause wide-ranging impacts on physical, mental, and emotional health.

The Adaptive Flexibility of the ANS

Each presentation underscores the remarkable adaptive flexibility of the ANS in meeting our needs for connection, activation, and shutdown in accordance with the safety or threat bias of our neuroception. Our nervous system is on our side.

Throughout the day, we seamlessly transition among the physiological states in response to cues from our environment. Detecting signals of safety reflexively prompts an autonomic shift toward the connected, ventral vagal state fostering feelings of calm, curiosity, and an openness to social connection. Conversely, cues signaling danger initiate a shift into a survival state—initially activating the sympathetic system and potentially leading to a submissive dorsal vagal state if the threat feels overwhelming. In states of fear or defense, we can't trust, we can't connect, and we can't heal.

Frequent shifts among physiologic states are important to acknowledge, as our current state serves as the foundational platform for all of our behavior. When danger cues outweigh safety signals, our availability and connection become compromised, impeding clear thinking as our body readies itself for defense. This imbalance can lead to misinterpretations of others' words, body language, and facial expressions, hindering our ability to perceive safety from those around us. Our state not only influences neuroception but also creates a feedforward loop where state begets state.

Autonomic Tendency

Each of us identifies with a personal autonomic tendency.[4] That is, when defensive, we are prone to shift into a particular survival state. Just reading this sentence, it's likely that your own autonomic tendency came straight to mind. You don't need to think hard about it: you either usually respond with the activation of fight or flight or by retreating into disconnection or shutdown. It's possible, maybe even likely, if your circumstances are particularly stressful, to become trapped in the cyclic defense loop where you oscillate continuously between a mobilized sympathetic state and an immobilized dorsal vagal state.

Understanding your own autonomic tendency is valuable because it allows you to recognize when you're in a particular state. This awareness helps you identify the triggers that led to that state and to know how to shift out of it, if appropriate.

We Are All Connected

Our autonomic state is the intervening variable, or mediator, between a stimulus in our world and our response to it. Simply put, our responses to life are dictated by the state we're in, yet we often react to events and people as if *they* are the cause of the way we feel. Recognizing that our state is a powerful intervening variable allows for increased awareness and understanding of our own and others' behaviors.

Viewing behavior through a polyvagal lens reveals that our behavior is influenced by our autonomic state rather than being a conscious choice. Reactions from others or ourselves—such as anger or apathy—can be viewed as signals of defense rather than deliberate blame or disregard. Responding to situations with a deeper sense of compassion and understanding of behavior—both our own and that of others—allows us to engage more empathetically and wisely. This is the forgiving aspect of PVT.

Furthermore, our states are contagious. Through facial expressions, vocal quality, body language, and energy, we unconsciously transmit our state to others. The other person's nervous system, in turn, intuitively gauges our demeanor and their own sense of safety through neuroception. Without our awareness, our nervous systems synchronize, reinforcing cues of threat or safety. Defensive states can initiate downward spirals. On the other hand, a ventral vagal state can propagate safety and connection.

The hopeful aspect of PVT is that the ANS, like the brain, can change. Our nervous system responses have been shaped by our habits and experiences, but these patterns are not fixed. They can be changed, and new ones can be created. Through our attention and intention, we can enhance our autonomic flexibility, opening up new possibilities for ourselves and those around us.

In any moment, we *are* our autonomic state because our state is the platform for all of our sensations, thoughts, emotions, and behaviors. The state of our ANS is influenced by the states of others', and likewise, we reciprocally affect theirs. Regardless of our differences in age, gender identity, sexual orientation, race, ethnicity, socioeconomic status, abilities, belief systems, or culture, we are all connected to each other through our nervous systems.

Strengthening Autonomic Resilience

Understanding the organization and tendencies of our individual nervous system is the first step to strengthening autonomic resilience. By recognizing the bodily sensations, thoughts, emotions, and behaviors associated with each of our physiological states, we become more attuned to our nervous system. As this awareness grows, we can actively engage in co-regulation and participate in regulating exercises and activities, fostering autonomic flexibility and resilience.

Repeated experiences of nervous system disruptions and subsequent repairs, whether through co-regulation or self-regulation, contribute to building autonomic resilience. With practice, we can guide our ANS toward safety and connection and relearn autonomic balance. Among other tools and approaches, SSP can help us gradually retune our autonomic responses, enhancing both fluidity and resilience.

Chapter 2

The Safe and Sound Protocol:
A Groundbreaking Polyvagal Approach

S SP is an innovative listening therapy based on PVT that can bring about transformational change. By using filtered music designed to elicit feelings of safety complemented by support from an attuned provider, SSP helps reset the ANS to its natural state supporting health, growth, restoration, and connection. Safety is the treatment, and sound is the vehicle. Though this may sound simple, the mechanisms driving these changes are quite complex and embedded in the intricacies of the ANS.

Exploring SSP and Its Impact

SSP is evidence-based and aims to facilitate balance and flexibility of the ANS. In peer-reviewed publications it has been documented to reduce auditory hypersensitivities, improve auditory processing, calm the ANS, and reduce symptoms of anxiety and depression. Collectively, these outcomes support social engagement and connection.

As a listening therapy, SSP uses music that has been specifically filtered to highlight the frequencies of the human voice. These sounds are cues of safety to the nervous system and stimulate the calming attributes of the parasympathetic nervous system. Within the frequency filtration algorithm, there are intervals when these safe sounds temporarily fade away before returning. This dynamic pattern serves as a neural exercise training autonomic capacity by intermittently engaging and disengaging the vagal brake. As this process repeats over time, it cultivates improved state regulation and fosters flexibility in the nervous system.

SSP works best when it is experienced with an attuned and supportive clinician who has been certified as an SSP provider since co-regulation is an important input to the process. A parent or close adult can also deliver SSP to a child if they are supervised by such a clinician. The relationship between the provider and the client is as important as the input of the sound.

Providers represent a wide variety of therapeutic disciplines. And because every client is unique, there is no single right way to deliver SSP. Nevertheless, certain consistent practices in SSP delivery have facilitated a positive experience for both the client and provider and have demonstrated efficacy. They are as follows:

- Getting to know each other at the start, setting the context, and confirming expectations for the experience of SSP

- Providing psychoeducation about the ANS through the lens of PVT so the client understands the role of the nervous system in their life experiences

- Exploring the client's unique nervous system and their autonomic tendencies

- Co-creating a shared language around the nervous system using metaphors, colors, and stories, which usually resonate better than scientific jargon

- Deciding together how to pace the listening and continually assessing the just-right titration of listening times

- Processing and integrating any physical or emotional sensations that arise during listening segments

- Reviewing the client's experience since the last session

- Continuously adapting the experience to match the client's needs as appropriate and continuously providing co-regulation

It's also important to understand what SSP is not. SSP is not a type of talk therapy. The client's narrative, while important, need not be a part of working with SSP. This makes it a refreshing approach for people who find talk therapy uncomfortable or ineffective. It also makes SSP suitable for people across a wide range of ages and abilities, including those with physical and cognitive challenges. While the client's story is not necessarily part of SSP delivery, the client's awareness of their visceral responses during SSP sessions is very helpful.

The provider modifies their facilitation based on the client, their situation, and their nervous system. SSP sessions can be conducted in-person or remotely depending on the client's comfort, convenience, and availability. The therapy involves listening to five hours of music but the experience of SSP delivery can range from two weeks to several months depending on the client's nervous system, their presenting features or symptoms, and the context of their life.

SSP is designed to be integrated with other therapeutic modalities but is also offered as a stand-alone experience. Providers are clinicians representing over 50 different professional disciplines, spanning from occupational and physical therapy to education, psychotherapy, psychology, somatic therapies, medicine, addiction counseling, ADHD coaching, speech and language therapy, bodywork, and more.

SSP sessions vary based on the provider's discipline. For example, occupational therapists, physical therapists, and bodyworkers may integrate SSP by having clients listen while engaging in light movement, receiving massage, or undergoing manual therapy. Psychologists and psychotherapists may use SSP to complement their ongoing therapeutic work. Teachers or learning specialists may introduce it to students during extracurricular programming. Providers often observe that SSP not only accelerates progress in other modalities, but it also facilitates access to new areas of therapy or learning. Clients may become more social, accessible, embodied, curious, and aware through the process of SSP delivery.

SSP sessions typically last an hour, during which the elements described above are incorporated based on the provider's therapeutic approach.

Within an SSP session, titrated SSP listening segments are included. Functionally, the client experiences SSP as a state modulator, helping them move toward an autonomic state of calmness and accessibility and away from a state of self-protective defensiveness. The client's neuroception reflexively dampens defense, dissipates feelings of stress and anxiety, and spontaneously moves toward a calm state that enhances spontaneous social engagement, creativity, curiosity, and cognitive function.

Because SSP works at the level of the brainstem's regulation of the ANS and doesn't rely on cognition, it's suitable for all people. Those who benefit from SSP often experience improvements in nervous system regulation and social engagement. Noticeable social enhancements include better vocal intonation, increased facial expressivity, greater eye contact, refined auditory processing, and improved co-regulation and connection.

These social improvements can positively impact other bodily systems regulated by the ANS such as the heart, breath, gut, metabolism, muscles, hormones, sleep, immunity, cognition, emotions, and energy, as described in chapter 1. Clients may notice a reduction in physical symptoms and relief from conditions associated with these systems. However, the primary aim of SSP delivery is to alleviate dysregulation. The polyvagal approach underlying SSP shifts the focus away from specific diagnoses or diseases to the sensations, thoughts, emotions, and behaviors associated with defensive states.

Clients who experienced SSP (and their parents, partners, and loved ones) have described the following overall improvements to their lived experience:

- Restored sense of belonging and connection in life
- New feelings of trust and generosity
- Increased spontaneity
- First hug from their child
- Enhanced and genuine connection to loved ones

- Ability to respond to challenges with openness rather than being triggered by them
- Greater self-compassion
- Less involvement in solitary play and more interest in playing with others
- Increased laughter and sense of humor
- Improved ability to interpret not only the words but the intent in conversations
- Renewed motivation
- Rejuvenating sleep and greater energy upon waking
- Expanded emotional availability
- Better self-awareness and embodiment
- Increased concentration
- Improved ability to express oneself authentically
- Greater capacity for co-regulation and relationship
- Restored interest in participating in life

The impact of SSP on our autonomic state—the intervening variable between stimulus and response—profoundly influences our reactions to the world and life events. When our ANS is fluid and we can move easily into a ventral vagal state, we become more open and less defensive. Things that would once have been irritating may now be less so. The murmurs of anxiety, agitation, or fear may be quieted. These positive shifts not only benefit the person receiving SSP but also extend to their family, friends, classmates, colleagues, and anyone they interact with.

SSP can initiate the process of feeling safe and accessible and open an opportunity to begin trusting that it's safe to feel safe again. This allows for greater openness, trust, rapport, and connection.

The Social Engagement System

Genuine, compassionate, emotional connections are a vital component to both physiological and mental health. Conversely, feeling defensive impedes social engagement, leading to isolation and loneliness. This not only harms our emotional well-being but also debilitates our overall health. When people feel isolated and disconnected, their health deteriorates, and there is a significant increase in depression and suicide rates. According to the US surgeon general, loneliness is an epidemic, with the impact of social isolation on our physiology comparable to smoking up to 15 cigarettes a day.[1]

The importance of social connection to humans traces back millions of years to our mammal, primate, and human ancestors. Social bonds form the foundation for our families and communities, unifying us through our cooperation rather than self-interest. Theodosius Dobzhansky, the prominent geneticist and evolutionary biologist, reflected this when he reframed the somewhat competitive narrative of "survival of the fittest" by suggesting that "the fittest may also be the gentlest, since survival often hinges on mutual help and cooperation."[2] Achieving mutual help and cooperation relies on an ANS capable of downregulating threat reactions and facilitating connection and collaboration. We evolved to feel safe and connect with others.[3]

PVT tells the story of how and when we can feel safe and connected. It describes social connectedness as a "biological imperative" for humans because our survival is dependent on trusted others. The development of the SES is evidence of this. A cluster of functions that spring from nerves emerging closely from the brainstem, the SES orchestrates our capacity to interpret and express social behaviors as appropriate. The interconnected nerves spark a chain reaction that can quickly light up one's face to express delight.

The SES is so important to our ability to thrive that it is already intact in full-term newborns. In utero, the glossopharyngeal nerve, along with the facial and trigeminal nerves, becomes part of the ventral vagal complex (elaborated on in chapter 3) and contributes to the quality and intonation of our voice. Voice is an essential indicator of our autonomic state, and it influences others' perceptions of us. When faced with threats, subtle alterations in our voice, like a harsh, shrill, or flat tone, unconsciously signal to those around us that we might be experiencing stress and may not be approachable. Conversely, when we feel safe and accessible, our voice reflects that too, with a soft and melodic tone, indicating our openness to connection.

The sound of our voice, the way we interpret speech, and how we're perceived are profoundly impacted by our own nervous system and those of others. Because of the significant role that voice and sound play in our capacity for connection, the auditory system—listening to music specifically—became the natural pathway for SSP.

The Use of Music

"Music, uniquely among the arts, is both completely abstract and profoundly emotional. It has no power to represent anything particular or external, but it has a unique power to express inner states or feelings. Music can pierce the heart directly; it needs no mediation,"[4] writes Oliver Sacks, the prominent British-American neurologist.

Research on music therapy supports its effectiveness in emotional, physical, cognitive, and social realms. A 2020 overview of research into music and stress suggests that listening to music can lower our heart rate and cortisol levels, release endorphins and improve our sense of well-being, distract us, reduce physical and emotional stress levels, and reduce stress-related symptoms, whether used in a clinical environment or in daily life.[5]

Music transcends mere auditory sensation; it embodies a shared experience that spans cultures, eras, and contexts. Whether pulsating in a drum circle, inspiring movement on the dance floor, resonating in a grand concert hall, or streaming through digital platforms, "music is a social symphony and offers a language that unites us."[6] From protest songs igniting social change to anthems evoking national pride, music has unified people around the world and across time. Likewise, communal singing—whether around a campfire or a karaoke machine—fosters a sense of camaraderie and belonging.

From a therapeutic perspective, music activates brain regions linked to reward, empathy, emotion, memory, and motivation, providing a wide array of advantages such as facilitating emotional expression and regulation, reducing stress, improving mood, and enhancing cognitive function. Importantly, it fosters social connection and cooperation, overcoming cultural and language differences to bring people together in profound ways that few other art forms can achieve.[7] SSP capitalizes on these therapeutic and socially engaging qualities by using music as its vehicle.

The Music of SSP

The music of SSP has two components: the underlying music playlist and the application of frequency filtration known as filtration pathways.

Music Playlists

There are multiple underlying music playlists of SSP ranging from classical, popular vocal, and fusion to children's music. Each music playlist is available in the three levels of filtration algorithms listed below, ensuring a consistent therapeutic experience regardless of which music playlist is chosen.

The choice of the underlying music playlist is individual, allowing users to select one based on their preferences. Playlists include a selection of pop and folk vocal tracks from the 1970s to the 1990s and an eclectic mix of instrumentals, pop rock, and rhythmic tunes. There is also a special playlist for children that includes songs from movies, nursery rhymes, and lullabies. Additionally, classical and fusion playlists are included, deliberately kept lyric-free to avoid any interference from words or meanings in the therapeutic experience. These universal playlists are designed to be inclusive, welcoming people of any age from all countries and cultures.

It's worth mentioning that the filtration process slightly alters the sound of the music, making it sound a bit distorted. Trained musicians may need to be warned of this because they will be especially aware of the music sounding slightly different from the artist's original presentation.

Filtration Pathways

There are three different filtration pathways, each with a different degree of filtration of the underlying music playlists. Which pathway—or degree of filtration—to choose is a key consideration in SSP delivery. The provider will make this decision together with their client taking into account their presenting needs, sensitivities, and the intensity of their features and symptoms. The three main filtration pathways are presented below in descending order of potency, ranging from therapeutic-level filtration to zero filtration.

SSP Core

SSP Core is the name given to the five hours of music with the original filtration algorithm. It is the most potent of the three pathways and is the topic of this book. Where you have read "SSP" thus far, it has referred specifically to SSP Core.

The underlying music is filtered through an algorithm that changes dynamically over the five hours. At the beginning, the filtration delivers a narrow band of frequencies associated with the frequencies of the human voice that the listener can receive regardless of their autonomic state or the neural tone of their auditory system. These sounds were chosen because they represent a distilled essence of safety.

As the music proceeds, the frequencies shift dynamically and progressively to train the neural network associated with listening. The range of the frequency band increases over the five hours, starting with the narrowest frequency band during Hour 1 and increasing to the widest frequency band during Hour 5. Additionally, within each hour, the frequency bands expand and contract, ranging from 200–5,000 Hz. This is considerably narrower than commercial music, which can range from 50–15,000 Hz.

SSP Balance

SSP Balance uses a lighter filtration algorithm with a slightly wider overall frequency band than SSP Core. Importantly, the filtration in SSP Balance does not progress dynamically across the five hours of music, which means it does not proactively challenge the neural network associated with listening. Practitioners use it to continue or extend the benefits of SSP after completing SSP Core and as an in-the-moment "state shifter" to soothe the nervous system. SSP Balance is overseen by an SSP provider, but the provider does not need to be present for the listening.

People use SSP Balance in various ways. Some parents play SSP Balance in the morning to reduce the stress of getting ready for school. Nervous flyers listen to it before and during flights. Others listen to it during dentist appointments. SSP Balance is also known to increase productivity and reduce procrastination.

SSP Connect

The music of the SSP Connect pathway is completely unfiltered and sounds just as it would on the radio or a streaming platform.

SSP Connect is sometimes used before SSP Core to give listeners familiarity with the music before any filtration, creating a sense of predictability by allowing them to know what comes next. Many people enjoy listening to SSP Connect after completing SSP Core because they grew fond of the underlying playlist and associate it with the calm and connected feelings they experienced during their initial sessions with SSP Core.

Although SSP Connect does not include any frequency filtration, unfiltered music has therapeutic benefits of its own. In an early study of SSP (then called the Listening Project Protocol), some child subjects were assigned to a control group who listened to the unfiltered versions of the playlist. While they did not experience the same degree of benefit as those in the experimental group, they did experience benefits in the areas of spontaneous speech (nonprompted use of language to communicate thoughts and ideas) and listening (the ability to understand spoken words without visual or contextual cues).[8]

SSP Is Different from Many Other Therapeutic Modalities

Many effective mental health therapies are top-down, meaning that they focus on cognitive processes like thoughts, beliefs, and emotions to influence well-being. They typically require active participation and engagement in the therapeutic process to build insight, self-awareness, and skills to make meaningful changes in the client's life. Some treatments use medications such as antidepressants or antipsychotics and medical procedures like transcranial magnetic stimulation or deep brain stimulation.

SSP uses a different approach. It retunes the ANS by delivering cues of safety through music and directly stimulating the SES. SSP may be conceptualized as a bidirectional, passive, noninvasive, acoustic vagus nerve stimulator. Understanding these concepts helps to better comprehend how SSP works.

SSP Recruits Both Top-Down and Bottom-Up Processes

Top-down (cognitive) approaches have a long history of prominence in mental health. Examples include cognitive behavioral therapy (CBT), dialectical behavior therapy (DBT), Acceptance and Commitment Therapy (ACT), psychodynamic therapy, and gestalt therapy.

With the integration of neuroscience into psychotherapy and a deeper understanding of the nervous system's role in mental health, there has been a growing interest in and adoption of bottom-up (somatic) approaches in contemporary therapeutic practices. These methods are particularly effective for individuals whose cognitive functioning may be compromised due to trauma, chronic defensiveness, illness, or disability. As described in chapter 1, in defensive states, the body does not prioritize executive functions or higher cognition, making top-down approaches less effective for some. Bottom-up approaches like biofeedback, Somatic Experiencing, Sensorimotor Psychotherapy, yoga therapy, and therapies focused on the client's bodily sensations and ANS are examples of approaches that leverage the complex interplay between the brain and body in mental health and wellness.

SSP delivery combines elements of both cognitive and somatic approaches to enhance the capacity of the nervous system. By working with a knowledgeable provider who provides psychoeducation about PVT, clients can better understand the effects of their autonomic state and their own unique autonomic tendencies. This is a top-down approach.

Listening to SSP itself is bottom-up as the sensory input of the filtered music is transmitted to the brainstem, engaging the body-brain connection. The co-regulation between the provider and client is also a bottom-up input as it involves visual cues as well as the nonverbal and the unconscious processes of neuroception and interoception.

Helping the client to experience their physiological states and the associated sensations, thoughts, emotions, and behaviors invites the understanding that these features are not necessarily under voluntary control but can be instead adaptive and reflexive outcomes of the ANS.[9] This involves both bottom-up and top-down pathways.

The Brainstem's Role in Connecting the Body and Brain

The brainstem, deep inside the brain, modulates subconscious vital bodily functions like heart rate, breath, temperature regulation, balance, reflexes, digestion, and sleep through the ANS. As the key intersection between the brain and the body, the brainstem serves as the integration and relay station for sensory (feeling) and motor (behavior) pathways, playing an important role in processing the level of our safety or threat and in allocating our resources and shifting our state.

Sensory information from the body is directed first to the brainstem, then to higher brain regions such as the thalamus, amygdala, and the prefrontal cortex. Multiple networks then assimilate and interpret these sensory experiences and visceral sensations. Informed by the signals in these networks, commands from the motor cortex travel downward to the brainstem and connect with nerves, organs, and muscles to initiate movement and behaviors.

Not just a relay station, the brainstem also integrates and modulates sensory and motor information to coordinate autonomic responses such as breathing, heart rate, and digestion. This is done through multiple feedback loops to manage our bodily resources and maintain homeostasis. These loops allocate resources toward physiological states of connection, activation, or shutdown.

Through the brainstem and feedback loops, the inputs of safety from the filtered SSP music and co-regulation with the provider generate effects on heart rate, breathing, and social engagement. The more cues of safety received in the brainstem, the more signals to calm the body are activated with the potential experience of openness, connection, and general well-being.

SSP Is a Passive Therapy

As a passive therapy, SSP allows access to the client's ANS without any active demand on their part. The frequency-filtered music provides a pattern of sounds to the nervous system that is unambiguously interpreted as signals of safety and accessibility. The sounds just come in and influence the ANS directly without any conscious awareness or physical process required of the client.

Other forms of passive input occur in our everyday lives as we are constantly taking in cues from the environment and other people. Facial expressions, body language, auditory signals, environmental context, and social and visual cues can all inform our sense of safety in the world.

Once in a safe state, the entire nervous system, including higher brain structures, becomes more available for further change from active approaches, including many therapeutic modalities and disciplines, such as psychotherapy, occupational therapy, dance, play, and movement therapies as well as breathwork, singing, chanting, yoga poses, and meditation, which we can do on our own.

By activating the vagus nerve and SES, SSP can support and enhance change from these and other approaches. In fact, both the effects of SSP and the other modality may be improved by their combination. In this way, changes from SSP can be cumulative and self-perpetuating.

SSP as a Noninvasive, Acoustic Vagal Nerve Stimulator

The SSP is aptly named and patented as an "acoustic vagus nerve stimulator" to distinguish it from traditional vagus nerve stimulation (VNS) devices. VNS devices are medical instruments designed to electrically stimulate the vagus nerve to produce therapeutic effects for conditions like epilepsy and treatment-resistant depression. Approval by the Food and Drug Administration in the US was granted in 1997 for the use of VNS for epilepsy and, in 2005, for depression. While early VNS devices were surgically implanted, recent innovations include noninvasive VNS that delivers the stimulation through the skin. A proliferation of noninvasive vagal nerve stimulators now exists to address a wide range of disorders such as migraines, anxiety, and inflammatory disorders.

VNS devices act as prostheses, artificially augmenting vagus nerve function for symptom reduction. However, unlike SSP, their effects are mostly temporary. When the VNS is turned off, so are the responses. A study on adolescents with functional abdominal pain disorders revealed that pain was reduced during VNS but returned upon the cessation of stimulation.[10]

While important for symptom reduction, there is little evidence that VNS devices can create long-term change or train the ANS to become more flexible and resilient. SSP Balance is similar to a standard VNS because it has a stable frequency band and does not proactively exercise the neural network associated with listening. It does, however, act as a temporary in-the-moment autonomic state shifter. Thus, although it may shift the user's autonomic state into a calmer, more welcoming ventral vagal state, the duration of the effect will be dependent on the resilience of the client's ANS at the time of use.

In contrast, SSP Core is designed as a neural exercise that enhances state regulation to improve resilience. Like a VNS, SSP Core stimulates the vagus nerve, but it does so through a more integrated challenge of the nervous system. The filtered music of SSP engages and disengages the vagal brake causing the listener's ANS to shift frequently between defensive states and a ventral vagal state. This movement increases the flexibility and capacity of the ANS. Improvements from SSP Core can be long-lasting and observed across various domains, including behavior, emotions, sensations, and physiology. SSP promotes resilience and flexibility for physiological state just as exercise does for muscles. Illnesses, injuries, or adverse experiences can temporarily disrupt these improvements, but providers have found that these gains can be restored through repeated exposure to SSP.

Laboratory and Peer-Reviewed Research Summary Through Charts, Tables, and Graphs

Below we summarize the research conducted on the Listening Project Protocol (LLPP) and SSP. The findings are outlined, with key insights presented in summary charts, tables, and graphs.

SSP Improves Auditory Processing[11]

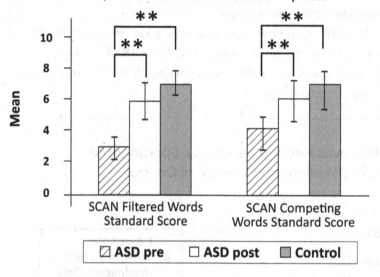

SCAN standard scores for ASD participants before and after intervention compared to performance of control participants. Error bars represent +/− two standard errors of the mean. ** = p < .01.

In a peer-reviewed study, autistic individuals who had lower support needs were tested using LPP, the precursor to SSP. Assessments included parent questionnaires, an auditory processing test, and heart rate monitoring. The study showed that auditory processing improved following the intervention.

Auditory processing, which had been highly compromised in the autism spectrum disorder (ASD) sample prior to the intervention, shifted to a level similar to the control group. Auditory processing was evaluated with the SCAN-3 Test for Auditory Processing Disorders (SCAN-3:C for children and SCAN-3:A for adults and adolescents). The SCAN-3 is a reliable assessment instrument used to evaluate auditory processing disorders. The two subscales—filtered and competing words—assessed the ability to focus on sounds and their meaning while filtering out competing auditory input. In research involving 33 people with

ASD aged 6 to 21 and 49 control participants aged 6 to 21, significant improvements in the ASD group were observed from before and after SSP. So much so that the ASD group post-SSP scores on the SCAN-3 subscales were no longer significantly different from the control group.

In addition, ventral vagal state regulation, measured by the amplitude of respiratory sinus arrhythmia (RSA), was tested. The study documented that vagal state regulation improved following the intervention.

SSP Improves Hearing Sensitivity, Spontaneous Speech, Listening, and Emotional Control[12]

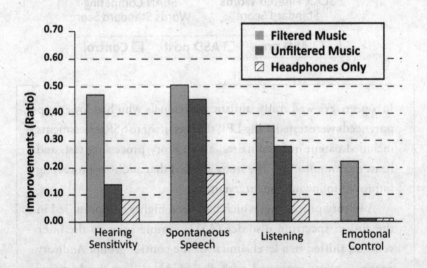

In a second peer-reviewed study, autistic children who used the LPP were evaluated in two trials. Trial 1 tested the difference between playing calmly while wearing headphones to listen to the specially treated music and while wearing headphones with no sound. Trial 2 tested the difference between using the intervention with the specially treated music and using it with untreated music. Despite being naive to which group their child was in, parents of the children who received the full intervention in each trial reported significant improvements in the domains of hearing sensitivities, listening, speech, and emotional control. The two-trial design helped researchers differentiate and contrast effects to the filtered music and the normal unfiltered music. The figure illustrates the composite data from the two trials.

As illustrated, listening to the filtered music selectively reduced auditory sensitivities and improved emotional control, while listening to either the filtered or the music without the filtering algorithm enhanced spontaneous speech and listening. Further evaluations documented that a subgroup of children who experienced a post-intervention improvement in hearing sensitivity also increased the amount of sharing behavior during a 10-minute semi-structured play-based protocol.

SSP Improves the Regulation of Hypersensitivities in Autistic People[13]

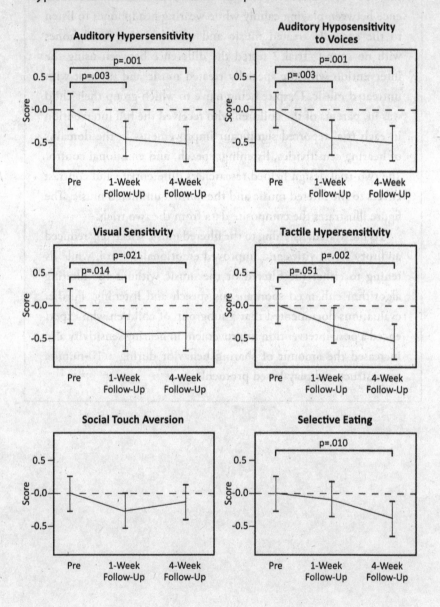

Auditory Hypersensitivity

p=.001

p=.003

0.5 –
Score
-0.0
-0.5 –

Pre | 1-Week Follow-Up | 4-Week Follow-Up

Auditory Hyposensitivity to Voices

p=.001

p=.003

0.5 –
Score
-0.0
-0.5 –

Pre | 1-Week Follow-Up | 4-Week Follow-Up

Visual Sensitivity

p=.021

p=.014

0.5 –
Score
-0.0
-0.5 –

Pre | 1-Week Follow-Up | 4-Week Follow-Up

Tactile Hypersensitivity

p=.002

p=.051

0.5 –
Score
-0.0
-0.5 –

Pre | 1-Week Follow-Up | 4-Week Follow-Up

Social Touch Aversion

0.5 –
Score
-0.0
-0.5 –

Pre | 1-Week Follow-Up | 4-Week Follow-Up

Selective Eating

p=.010

0.5 –
Score
-0.0
-0.5 –

Pre | 1-Week Follow-Up | 4-Week Follow-Up

This is the first study to assess the effects of SSP on auditory, visual, and tactile sensitivities and selective eating, as well as being the first ASD-specific study of SSP in Germany. The study involved delivery of SSP to 37 autistic children and adults. Results from the Brain-Body Center Sensory Scales (BBCSS) demonstrated reduced auditory hypersensitivity, hyposensitivity to the human voice, and visual hypersensitivity at the one-week and four-week follow-up assessments. Tactile hypersensitivity and selective eating showed significant decline at the four-week follow-up assessment.

SSP Improves Measures of Autonomic Reactivity, Anxiety, and Depression[14]

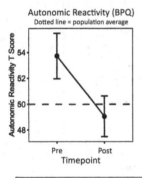
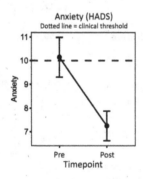
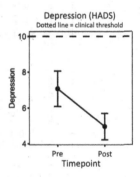

The Body Perception Questionnaire Short Form, a scale developed by the Porges laboratory, and the Hospital Anxiety and Depression Scale (HADS) were administered to 33 clients with voice, throat, and breathing problems pre- and post-SSP. A significant decrease was found in all of the subscales. Not only did SSP reduce symptoms of anxiety and depression and affect the functioning of the ventral vagal complex as indicated by the reduction in scores on the supra-diaphragmatic subscale, but there was also a reduction in the symptoms expressed in organs regulated by the dorsal vagus. Together, these results suggest that participants experienced enhanced autonomic and emotional regulation following SSP.

SSP Improves Social Engagement Behaviors and Physical Movement and Supports the Reduction of Symptoms of Functional Neurological Disorder[15]

Pre- and Post-Treatment Measures of the Depression, Anxiety, and Stress Scales (DASS) and the Body Perception Questionnaire (BPQ)

	Measure & Domain	Pre-SSP	1 Month Post-SSP
		Clinical Range	Normal Range
Depression, Anxiety & Stress Scales	Depression Scale	18	2
	Anxiety Scale	21	1
	Stress Scale	17	8
	Total DASS Score	56	11

		Clinical Range	Normal Range
Body Perception Questionnaire	Body Awareness (T-score)	63.4	42
	Supradiaphragmatic Reactivity (T-Score)	70.6	43.7
	Subdiaphragmatic (Gut) Reactivity (T-Score)	72.8	36.6

In a case study published by the *Harvard Review of Psychiatry*, a child with functional neurological disorder who was unresponsive to other treatments had a transformative response to SSP. Notably, her social engagement improved alongside significant enhancements in physical mobility. These improvements included the cessation of wheelchair use, a return to a normalized gait, and regained abilities to climb and engage in play.

As illustrated in the table, the pre-SSP levels for anxiety and depression moved from clinically concerning to normal. Moreover, on the Body Perception Questionnaire, her levels of body awareness and autonomic reactivity moved from being clinically concerning to within the normal range.

SSP Decreases Hyperarousal, Negative Mood, and Cognitive Symptoms[16]

In a currently unpublished pilot study, clients diagnosed with PTSD were administered trauma-informed psychotherapy either with SSP (19 participants) or without SSP (12 participants). The results document that the use of SSP as an adjunctive therapy enhanced clinical outcomes resulting in statistically significant symptom improvement profiles. Specifically, during the one-week follow-up, the SSP group reported greater improvement on total PTSD symptoms compared to the therapy-only group (13.67 versus 2.50, $p<.05$). Post hoc analyses showed that group differences were driven by decreases in hyperarousal ($p<.01$) and negative mood and cognition ($p <.05$) but not reexperiencing or avoidance symptoms. All significant effects (total PTSD symptoms, hyperarousal, and negative mood and cognition) persisted to the four-week follow up. Clients reported good acceptance of SSP. Seventy-five percent reported that they believed it helped achieve treatment goals, and 87.4 percent looked forward to the listening sessions.

Real-World Evidence

Real-world evidence (RWE) uses data collected outside of traditional clinical trials and controlled experiments, such as medical records, patient registries, and even health apps on your phone. This data helps us to better understand how treatments work and if they're safe to use in everyday life. RWE offers several advantages over clinical trials. It reflects real-world behavior, includes larger and more diverse participant groups, and provides faster results. However, it also has limitations, such as less control over variables and potential bias.

Unyte Health collects RWE through online assessments taken by clients of SSP providers. The data represents how clients respond to SSP services in real-world settings, but it doesn't control for other treatments or individual factors that might influence the outcomes. Clients of SSP providers have access to several online assessments on the Unyte Health dashboard. The choice of assessment is suggested by the provider, and the completion of the assessments by the client is voluntary. Once entered, the data is anonymized, removing the identifying details of personal information.

Unlike laboratory and clinical studies, this data does not represent matched sampling with controls or selective sampling based on clinical condition or history. This data represents the impact on clients who have elected to experience SSP with a provider who delivers SSP within their treatment model. Most providers use SSP as an adjunctive therapy. The data represents client response changes after completing the five-hour SSP program. Note that the duration of completing the five-hour program may vary greatly and that the clients may be receiving additional therapeutic support.

The assessments reported reflect symptoms associated with a diagnosis and do not in themselves constitute a diagnosis. Clients presenting to SSP providers with mental health symptoms are frequently encouraged to complete the frequently used symptom assessment instruments based on the Diagnostic and Statistical Manual of Mental Disorders (DSM-5) for anxiety (General Anxiety Disorder-7, or GAD-7), depression (Patient Health Questionnaire-9, or PHQ-9), and post-traumatic stress disorder (PTSD Checklist-5, or PCL-5). The caregivers of children who present with challenged psychosocial functions are encouraged to complete the frequently used Pediatric Symptom Checklist (PSC).

The RWE was consistent with clinical trials and laboratory research. All assessments documented reductions in symptoms with 80 to 90 percent of the clients reporting improvement. Perhaps even more encouraging was the impact on those whose scores suggested clinical concern. For this subgroup, approximately half no longer had a symptom profile suggesting concern.

Real-World Evidence

Assessment	Function	Sample Size	Improved	Clinical → Non-clinical	T-value	Significance Level
GAD-7	Anxiety	313	86%	61%	21.8	p<.00001
PHQ-9	Depression	208	81%	54%	10.7	p<.00001
PCL-5	PTSD	120	91%	63%	13.7	p<.00001
PSC	Psychosocial Function	94	83%	47%	8.0	p<.00001

A relative newcomer to the therapy world, SSP has proven to be very effective in addressing symptoms and features related to autonomic dysregulation by introducing essential safety into the nervous system. SSP integrates easily into many disciplines and can improve readiness for and enhanced progress in other modalities. As many peer-review studies, clinical trials, and case studies have demonstrated, whether used independently or as a complement to other approaches, SSP contributes to improving the flexibility and adaptability of the ANS, an essential element of both mental and physical well-being.

Chapter 3

How the Safe and Sound Protocol Works

Based on PVT and developed to improve autonomic regulation and enhance the connection between people, SSP works by infusing a *distilled essence of safety* into the client's nervous system. This is the first step toward any healing.

PVT demonstrates that our ability to survive and thrive is dependent on managing our physiological state via social connection. A quintessential example of this, though not one that everyone has experienced, is the profound bond between a mother and her baby and the extraordinary connection that unfolds as they become locked in each other's presence. Each one's gaze, movement, and energy are intricately synchronized with the other as they co-regulate. Their tangible connection highlights the bidirectionality of social interaction. The mother is not only regulating the infant, the infant is reciprocally regulating the mother as well. Engagement like this contributes to the emotional well-being and physical health of both mother and child.

This feeling of trust and safety can be conveyed through sounds, like a mother's lullaby. SSP may not reproduce the intimate bond of a mother and child, but the cues of safety it offers present a valuable alternative and a significant beginning for establishing trust.

Why SSP Is Effective

Insufficient research has been conducted to fully understand all of SSP's mechanisms of action. However, its efficacy can be explained through the concepts and principles of PVT, which we will delve into here. Additionally, we will explore how SSP effects changes within specific systems and hypothesize about the contribution of other systems and functions to the experiences of SSP providers and their clients.

One of the great aspects about SSP is that clients don't need to fully understand *how* it works *for* it to work. What's most important is that clients remain present in the moment with their provider and establish a meaningful connection together. However, for those who are curious, this chapter provides an explanation of SSP's underlying mechanisms.

SSP Retunes the ANS

While listening to SSP, the client's vagal brake is engaged and disengaged, facilitating movement along the autonomic continuum as the filtered music's frequency presentations shift. These dynamic frequency changes offer numerous opportunities to experience a connected ventral vagal state and to return there from a defensive state. This practice of moving through the continuum improves fluidity and flexibility, gradually reorganizing and fine-tuning the ANS and enhancing the ability to return to homeostasis more easily after a challenge.

This process builds and reinforces neuronal connections in the nervous system through myelinated pathways. Myelin, the fatty coating of axons (the nerve cell fibers that transmit electrical signals), not only speeds up signal transmission within a neural network but also ensures smoother and more efficient communication.

The neural networks of the ANS are strengthened by their very activation. By repeatedly practicing moving along the autonomic continuum using the vagal brake and thereby re-regulating, we are reinforcing the neuronal connections. Exercising the nervous system in this way strengthens autonomic flexibility and resilience.

Even beyond completion of SSP, the nervous system sustains and strengthens these new patterns of autonomic flexibility. As one navigates the world and engages socially, auditory input and neuroception continue to play pivotal roles. When cues of safety or threat, conveyed through the voices of people and the sounds in the environment, align with the feelings of safety or danger from those relationships and surroundings, the nervous system continues to retune by shifting along the autonomic continuum accordingly.

The Power of Co-Regulation

Co-regulation is the reciprocal supportive relatedness between people (and animal companions) that is facilitated by the activation of the SES. It is fueled by the genuine mutual affiliation between people who engage with each other in a positive and supportive manner. In such relationships, each person feels valued, heard, and in synchrony with the other.

Words are not needed for co-regulation. As noted earlier, babies can feel the connection without using language and so can the rest of us. The signals from one person's nervous system to another's are visceral and reciprocated, activating a physiology of connection through the ventral vagal complex. When we have one or more co-regulating relationships, we feel safe and connected. This experience gives us the capacity to self-regulate when we are on our own.

The attuned presence of a compassionate provider and the filtered music of SSP are each powerful elements of co-regulation. Together, there is a multiplying effect.

Engaging the SES

Our physiology includes a bidirectional communication circuit between the body and the brain, with the brainstem serving as its hub. It is from the brainstem—specifically, the ventral vagal complex—that the ventral pathway of the vagus nerve, our calming neural pathway, connects with four other cranial nerves (CNs) to form the SES. The five cranial nerves involved in the SES are the trigeminal nerve (CN V), facial nerve (CN VII), glossopharyngeal nerve (CN IX), vagus nerve (CN X), and accessory nerve (CN XI).

This group of nerves is involved in the innervation of the muscles of the head, face, ears, throat, heart, and lungs. When you have a warm encounter with a friend, and your and their facial expressions and voices are enlivened with the pleasure of connecting with each other, it is the cranial nerves of the SES creating this response.

These nerves contain both afferent (sensory) and efferent (motor) pathways that affect our social, emotional, and physical functions. Afferent pathways travel from the body to the brain, relaying information about the status of the body and neuroception to the ventral vagal complex and whether to increase or decrease vagal outflow to affect the system. Based on that information, efferent pathways travel from the brain to the body to regulate social engagement behaviors, including vocalizing, listening, adopting facial expressions, tilting the head, and regulating the heart and lungs.

When afferent sensory signals from the body to the brainstem convey safety, the ventral vagal complex responds by promoting increased vagal outflow and access to a ventral vagal state. This physiological shift results in reduced hypersensitivity to sounds, better perception of the human voice, enhanced facial expressivity (producing a genuine smile marked by wrinkles at the corners of the eyes), a rich, melodic voice, smooth breathing, slower heart rate, availability for companionship, and feelings of belonging and accessibility. Conversely, when we experience a neuroception of danger, these positive changes are reversed. Our face becomes less friendly, our auditory perception of human speech diminishes, our voice changes, and our overall demeanor conveys that we are not accessible. This dynamic forms a feedback loop where our physiology informs our SES, and our SES, in turn, impacts our physiology. Understanding this interplay highlights the intricate relationship between our physiological state and social behavior, emphasizing the importance of a supportive environment in maintaining autonomic balance.

The Impact of Sounds and Listening on the Autonomic State

Every one of the target organs of the SES provides a portal to activate the ventral vagal complex, but the auditory system was chosen for SSP because of the accessibility of acoustic input and our innate affinity, shared among social mammals, to calm in response to melodic vocalizations.

Sound Frequencies and the ANS

The ANS reacts to qualities of sound as signals of safety, neutrality, or threat. Within the continuum of audible sound waves, different frequency ranges provide different information to our nervous system, much like channels on a radio dial. Low frequencies tend to signal danger (think of the booming sound of thunder, the roar of a lion, or the vibrations of an earthquake) while high frequencies convey urgency and alert (consider alarms, ambulance sirens, screams, or a baby's high-pitched sounds of distress).[1] The middle range of sound frequencies, such as those of a female vocalist or a mother singing a lullaby to her baby, is where the sounds of a welcoming human voice reside.

Our earliest experiences of sound occur in utero during the second trimester. The predominant sounds are those of our mother's heartbeat and voice. By six month's gestation, we detect the prosody of her voice—that is, the rhythm, intonation, and musicality of her speech. Her voice becomes our earliest, most salient sound, and it brings us comfort and pleasure.[2] Once we are born, our sense of connection and regulation from our caregivers is essential—so much so that it can be called bio-logically imperative. Among other systems, our response to prosody contributes to our sense of safety and our ability to form relationships.

Research underscores the crucial role of caregiver voices to young ner-vous systems. Specifically, the middle frequencies (approximately 1,500 to 3,500 Hz) of a mother's or guardian's voice, alongside the prosody of their speech, are linked to reduced infant distress and improved autonomic reg-ulation following a stressor.[3] Additionally, the level of infant autonomic regulation correlates with the prosodic qualities of the mother's voice, which in turn adapts in response to the infant's distress cues.

Tuning In to Frequencies with the Middle Ear Muscles

The nervous systems of all social mammals, not just humans, have a special affinity for prosody, and our ears are equipped with structures capable of tuning in to the sounds of vocalizations and intonation. The smallest muscles in the body, the middle ear muscles, do the work of tuning our auditory perception in to different frequency ranges. When these muscles are tensed, they stiffen the chain of small bones in the middle ear called the ossicles. This action stretches the eardrum and optimizes the frequencies of the human voice to be transmitted through the auditory nerve to the cortex where it is processed. While these midrange frequencies are perceived by the brain, the lower frequency sounds bounce off the taut eardrum and are dampened.[4]

Metaphorically, the eardrum functions like the skin of a kettle drum, the tightness of which determines the frequencies the drum can produce. The tighter the skin, the higher the frequency. Percussionists use the drum's pedal to tighten or loosen the drum's skin and adjust its pitch. Similarly, in the eardrum, our autonomic state, facilitated by the ventral vagal complex, dynamically adjusts the activation of our middle ear muscles—specifically the tensor tympani and stapedius muscles, which are controlled by the CN V and the CN VII nerves—to regulate the tension of the eardrum, allowing it to respond dynamically to different sounds and frequencies.

When we are in a connected ventral vagal state, the middle ear muscles tighten, stretching the eardrum and allowing softer, higher-pitched sounds to pass through the middle ear structures into the inner ear and then through the auditory nerve to the brain. This enhances the perception of frequencies present in human voices. Music and voices containing the frequencies of the human voice can promote a natural shift into a ventral vagal state.

In autonomic states of defense, the middle ear muscles—and consequently the eardrum—relax, allowing louder low- and high-frequency sounds associated with danger and alarm to pass through, while filtering out the frequencies of the human voice. The ambient background noise of low and high frequencies in our environment can obscure the voices of those with whom we interact, potentially worsening a defensive state.

This is the experience of individuals whose middle ear muscles do not function properly, or whose ability to accurately tune in to the frequencies of the human voice is otherwise compromised. Several common factors may contribute to the dysfunction of the middle ear muscles:

- Ear infections can lead to the accumulation of fluid in the middle ear, which is typically an air-filled space. This fluid buildup can cause discomfort and hinder the contraction of the middle ear muscles. Reduced muscle function can also interfere with fluid drainage through the eustachian tubes, perpetuating a cycle of chronic ear infections and resulting in further immobility of the middle ear muscles.

- People with overall reduced muscle tone may also experience reduced middle ear muscle tone. This condition, known as hypotonia, is often linked to various medical conditions and disorders, such as Down syndrome, Ehlers-Danlos syndrome, hypermobility spectrum disorders, Prader-Willi syndrome, autism spectrum disorder, and muscular dystrophy.

- Trauma, which can induce chronic defensiveness, may prompt an adaptive recalibration of the middle ear muscles, prioritizing their responsiveness to lower- or higher-frequency sounds over the sounds of the human voice.

- Individuals with Bell's palsy experiencing paralysis of the facial nerve, including the branch that regulates the stapedius (a middle ear muscle regulating ossicle chain tension and the eardrum), report hyperacusis and struggle to discern speech amid background sounds.

Over time, immobility of the middle ear muscles resulting from any one of these factors may lead to "learned disuse" of the middle ear muscles and may trigger an adaptive retuning of the entire SES. However, with SSP it is possible to rehabilitate the middle ear muscles and reorient them to the frequencies of the human voice.

SSP Rehabilitates and Strengthens the
Capacity to Perceive Voices

As mentioned in the description of SSP Core in chapter 2, the filtration of the underlying music of SSP begins in the first hour by isolating and delivering only a narrow set of frequencies within the range of the human voice. Being the sole input, these distilled cues of safety are initially received directly by the auditory cortex regardless of the status of the middle ear muscles.

Some listeners may not have experienced safe sounds for a long time. Young children who have had ear infections or are on the autism spectrum often respond with delight to these soothing sounds, and the positive effect on their overall demeanor is immediately apparent.

For others, particularly those individuals who have been betrayed by someone they trusted, safe sounds can evoke feelings of vulnerability. For them, signals of safety might be perceived as threats, and their nervous system might adaptively respond to signals of safety by triggering a neuroception of vulnerability. Consequently, individuals with a history of severe adversity may initially only tolerate very short exposures to the filtered music. Their SSP provider will carefully monitor their response and titrate their exposure accordingly.

As the music progresses, the filtration expands and contracts around the frequency range of the human voice. At times, sounds in these frequencies are sufficiently dampened to become incomprehensible, only to return later. This variation exercises the middle ear muscles and may lead to exhaustion. Many SSP clients report that they or their child slept deeply following an SSP session. Since the middle ear muscles are fast-twitch muscles, they tend to fatigue rapidly, which can have a generalized effect on the body.

The neural exercise embedded in SSP is modulated to account for this. Like an athlete on a treadmill gradually increasing the elevation, speed, and time to challenge and improve muscle groups, the progressively filtered music ensures that the delivery of SSP doesn't overstrain, overwhelm, or exhaust the client's nervous system.

By the end of SSP Core, the client can perceive human voice frequencies even in the presence of the full range of sound. This capacity continues to be strengthened even after completing SSP, as engaging with others in a world of full-spectrum sound provides ongoing exercise for the middle ear muscles.

Autonomic State and Auditory Processes Are Improved by SSP

Strengthening the capacity to better perceive voices has a rehabilitative effect on the ANS. Being able to hear the full range of frequencies enables us to perceive subtle differences in pitch and tone, as well as the nuances of speech, including which words are stressed. With this auditory acuity, the meaning, emotion, and intention behind the words can be comprehended. This includes irony, humor, sarcasm, tone, and other social cues that may have been missed previously.

Hearing words correctly relies on the frequencies of human speech. Consonant sounds typically have higher frequencies (in the 1,000 to 4,000 Hz range). If these frequencies are dampened due to the state of the ANS or problems in the ear, many consonants (particularly *s, f, sh, th*, and *z*) will be difficult to perceive. Since consonants are often at the end of words and are less emphasized, this can lead to difficulties in differentiating words, following directions, and understanding speech clearly.

Misinterpreting the meaning of others is quite alienating and can disrupt communication. This is the experience of many people with a downregulated SES due to developmental trauma, PTSD, autism, anxiety, depression, or other causes of autonomic dysregulation.

A ventral vagal state not only contributes to better perception of speech sounds and auditory processing, but it may also reduce auditory hypersensitivities. These hypersensitivities can cause discomfort, pain, reduced noise tolerance, emotional distress, and even social isolation. Stress, anxiety, and depression can amplify the perception of loudness and discomfort, but with balanced autonomic regulation, hypersensitivities can be reduced.

Each of the four elements of the auditory functions—acoustic properties of sound, autonomic state, auditory processing, and auditory hypersensitivity—can interact with the ANS, and they can all positively influence one another. This creates a synergistic relationship where improvements in one factor may lead to enhancements in the others.

Evolutionarily, the ability to reduce background noise and focus on specific frequencies related to social communication was crucial for mammals to identify members of their own species. In modern times, tuning in to each other's voices plays a vital role in the neuroception of safety, autonomic state, auditory processing, and reduction of hypersensitivities.

The Effect of SSP on Specific Systems

While not directly researched, other biological mechanisms, including signaling responses, systems involving the cortical and midbrain areas along with the endocrine, immune, neuropeptide, sensory, and limbic systems, inflammatory processes, neurotransmitters, muscles, fascia, and the gut, are likely involved in the changes observed from SSP. This broad perspective is supported by current neuroscience research documenting neural pathways connecting the brain and nervous system to all bodily structures and functions. We hope this will encourage clinicians and academics to explore SSP further.

In this book, our focus is the ANS and PVT. Through the lens of these frameworks, we aim to provide a plausible explanation for the potential influence of SSP across various domains where observable changes frequently occur.

Each functional system described below has traditionally been viewed as being dependent on disparate neural circuits, but in fact they are all interconnected through the ANS and physiological state. SSP optimizes these systems and functions by recruiting the brainstem regulatory circuit of the ventral vagal complex. Specifically, SSP presents an acoustic pattern that neuroception detects as signals of safety, downregulating threat reactions. In this way, the sounds are literally giving permission to the nervous system to give up its defenses and enable accessibility, co-regulation, and sociality.

Sensory Systems

There is a strong relationship between autonomic state and sensitivities to sound, light, and touch. This connection is well-known within the autism community, among people who have experienced trauma, those with anxiety, and others who are drawn to SSP for the hope and relief it offers.

When the ANS enters a defensive state, the functional capacity of the ventral vagal complex is reduced, compromising social engagement behaviors such as biasing the interpretation of the intention of vocalizations. In survival-oriented autonomic states, the vagal regulation of heart rate and sensory systems geared toward social cues is suppressed and replaced by heightened sensitivity to threat signals. This lowers sensory thresholds across tactile, visual, and auditory domains, diminishing the ability to discern cues of accessibility and social interaction. Such blunting of the SES is a central feature of many mental health conditions and behavioral challenges.

By influencing the ventral vagal complex, SSP calms autonomic state and dampens hypersensitivities across several domains. SSP has reliably reduced hypersensitivities like those associated with autism and complex trauma as well as more specific sensitivities such as misophonia. The primary effects of SSP on the sensory system are achieved by calming autonomic state and engaging the middle ear muscles to enhance the signal-to-noise ratio between the sound of the human voice and background sounds. In addition, SSP induces a general increase in parasympathetic activation, which can influence sensory systems like vision. This leads to pupillary constriction and a reduction in visual hypersensitivity.

Cognitive Functioning

Autonomic state influences cognitive function. We all have had the experience of our higher thinking being unavailable to us in times of stress, making it more difficult to retrieve the names of people and objects or specific words. For example, if you are running late, it's difficult to remember where your keys are. Or when you have a health issue, you may struggle to remember your questions or the doctor's responses, even though they are of utmost importance. As story-making humans, we create a narrative about our lapses without recognizing that they are caused by temporary shifts in our physiological state. When a defensive state becomes chronic, it's understandable that we have reduced access to executive functions and higher cognition.

An early SSP case exemplifies this. Prior to undergoing SSP, a young boy scored an IQ of 70, but a month after completing SSP, his IQ test yielded a score of 140. It's not that SSP boosted his IQ but rather, by calming his ANS, his cognitive abilities could be more accurately assessed.

Survival is the brain's top priority. When the foundational brainstem survival circuits are recruited in defense, cognitive functioning in the cortex is diminished. This tradeoff between adaptive survival and cognitive function becomes evident when memory retrieval, decision-making, attentional focus, and problem-solving are impaired by feelings of threat. Conversely, a calm ventral vagal state engages higher brain circuits, enhancing problem-solving tasks such as sustained attention and memory retrieval. This state fosters creativity, insights, and flow.

Emotional Regulation

The areas of the brain that process and experience emotions, memories, and sensations are located above the brainstem areas that regulate autonomic state. When the brainstem areas regulating the ANS are locked into supporting survival, all neural circuits above the brainstem can be influenced, resulting in emotions such as fear, frustration, sadness, anger, and anxiety.

As SSP recruits brainstem areas that calm, the neural circuits above these foundational areas become accessible so that a more complex tapestry of emotions representing a broad range of feelings and associated memories may be experienced, especially for those with underlying trauma and attachment disorders.

When this occurs, qualified clinicians need to act with compassionate care to help the client acknowledge, express, and integrate these memories and feelings. Then the client can experience a whole new trajectory, bringing joy, hope, and previously unavailable opportunities to their life.

Chronic Pain

Chronic pain needs to be distinguished from acute pain, which is an adaptive reaction of the nervous system to injury or illness through identifiable pain receptors known as nociceptors. These nerve cell endings that detect damaging stimuli and send signals to the brain are located in the skin, deep tissues, and most visceral organs, ready to respond to chemical, mechanical, and thermal stimuli. Acute pain is due to the detection of a damaging stimulus similar to the pain of getting burned when touching something too hot. Medical interventions are highly effective for acute pain.

Most chronic pain, unlike acute pain, is not driven by a specific sensory pathway and is less responsive to pharmaceutical or other medical interventions. Instead, chronic pain results from a nervous system locked in a cyclic defense loop, where signals of danger persist even though the original source of the danger is no longer present. In essence, chronic pain reflects a nervous system that continues to receive signals from sensory pathways as if the damage is still occurring. Due to this mechanism, SSP may be helpful in reducing chronic pain.

Similar to other defense mechanisms, chronic pain is linked to dysregulation of the ANS, which is metabolically costly and often associated with increased heart rate, disrupted digestion, and heightened generalized inflammation. SSP, by recruiting the ventral vagal complex, downregulates the survival states of the nervous system. This process can restore balance, reduce inflammation, and transform the sensations and related emotions of chronic pain to a more manageable level.

Immune, Endocrine, and Neuropeptide Functions

The immune system partners with the ANS. In fact, PVT posits that there is an "expanded" ANS that includes endocrine, immune, and neuropeptide (e.g., oxytocin and vasopressin) functions.[5] Thus, when the ANS shifts into a state of threat, neurochemicals such as inflammatory cytokines, adrenalin, cortisol, and vasopressin are released to maintain the defensive state.

By recruiting the ventral vagal complex and the SES, SSP not only calms the ANS but also the "partner" neurochemical systems that support the homeostatic processes of health, growth, restoration, and sociality. The consequence of this coordinated activity supports healing from chronic illness and chronic inflammatory conditions.

There have been reports by SSP providers of major reductions in the symptoms associated with Long COVID, autoimmune diseases, and chemical sensitivities. Dr. Sue Carter, the scientist who discovered the relationship between oxytocin and social bonding, has speculated that the effectiveness of SSP in promoting a calmness in the ANS may also be related to the initiation of a neurochemical cascade resulting in the release of oxytocin.

Life's stressors can dysregulate the nervous system, manifesting in various symptoms as our body copes to ensure survival. Even *anticipating* harm can shift our ANS into a defensive state. These protective responses may trap us in a defensive cycle, hindering our well-being and social connections. But because the influence of the ANS is so extensive, SSP is associated with broad enhancements in physical, emotional, and mental health. By retuning our ANS toward optimal regulation, SSP initiates a positive cycle of transformation and opens new possibilities.

Chapter 4

Self-Directed Change and Healing: Retuning the Nervous System

S SP is just one of hundreds, if not thousands, of effective therapeutic approaches available to support the process of change and healing. These approaches range from ancestral to modern and Eastern to Western traditions, encompassing well-established top-down modalities like cognitive behavioral therapy and dialectical behavior therapy, as well as bottom-up approaches like Somatic Experiencing, Sensorimotor Psychotherapy, and biofeedback. Additionally, there are numerous specialized and niche approaches, including equine therapy, art therapy, and mindfulness techniques. Because SSP can enhance our ANS's flexibility and capacity, it can complement and enhance many of these therapeutic approaches.

We're currently witnessing a golden age of therapy because of increased awareness, research, societal acceptance of mental health issues, and advancements in technology making therapy more widely accessible. With the guidance of a well-matched therapist, one can gain insight into challenges, develop coping strategies, enhance self-understanding, improve relationships, and overcome obstacles. A crucial component of successful therapy is a safe and trusting relationship with the therapist.

All Healing Begins with Safety

From a polyvagal perspective, all healing begins with a sense of safety, which promotes a balanced and adaptable ANS. The ANS is crucial for our well-being, continuously working within us to manage our physiological responses to the environment. When we feel safe, our potential expands. By centering ourselves and seeking equilibrium, we initiate a positive feedback loop that guides our nervous system toward a state conducive to connection, change, and healing. By tapping into the natural support of our ANS, we make meaningful healing possible.

Alternatives to Formal Therapy

There are numerous free or inexpensive ways to foster safety and promote well-being. These include participating in yoga classes at local recreation centers, joining community choirs or drum circles, practicing tai chi or qigong in group settings, engaging in book clubs or support groups, attending group therapy sessions, joining meet-up groups for outdoor activities like hiking, volunteering in the community, and participating in topic-specific groups on social media platforms. Additionally, many in the therapeutic community offer free events and group activities, including webinars and online resources accessible from anywhere in the world.

In this chapter we present many activities and exercises that you can do on your own or with others to increase the flexibility and balance of your nervous system. They can be found in the "Regulation Toolbox" section, which contains three charts of suggested activities, one chart for each of the three primary physiological states. Small steps matter, as even incremental improvements in nervous system flexibility can profoundly impact well-being.

Upward Spirals: Small Steps Lead to Long-Term Change

Being in a ventral vagal state is not only pleasant but also more metabolically efficient for our nervous system. It promotes health and provides a neural foundation for peace and contentment. As one spends more time in a ventral vagal state it becomes easier to access, which creates a positive feedback loop described in these pages as "state begets state" and leads to upward spirals of well-being.

Researchers Bethany Kok and Barbara Frederickson[1] propose a reciprocal relationship between vagal tone and psychological well-being. They posit that vagal tone encourages individuals to actively engage in social and emotional opportunities that increase connectedness and positive emotions and lead to further increases in vagal tone. This "upward spiral" underscores how even brief positive experiences can accumulate over time, building personal recourses that significantly enhance overall well-being.

Consider the following example of an upward spiral. It illustrates how small, incremental steps can lead to lasting changes:

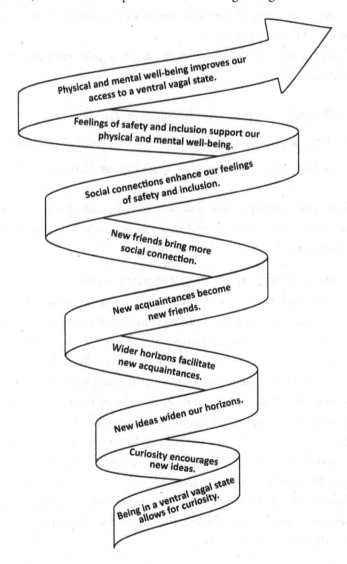

Physical and mental well-being improves our access to a ventral vagal state.

Feelings of safety and inclusion support our physical and mental well-being.

Social connections enhance our feelings of safety and inclusion.

New friends bring more social connection.

New acquaintances become new friends.

Wider horizons facilitate new acquaintances.

New ideas widen our horizons.

Curiosity encourages new ideas.

Being in a ventral vagal state allows for curiosity.

Preparatory Steps to Support Your Regulation Practice

Engaging in activities that regulate the nervous system and promote access to a ventral vagal state is a way to enhance vagal tone. There are numerous practical exercises you can do alone or with a friend to reset and rebalance your ANS. These exercises are convenient, adaptable to any setting, and require minimal time commitment. By investing just a few minutes regularly, you can significantly improve your ability to regulate and foster connection.

To begin, consider these preparatory steps to guide your choice of the activities and timing:

1. Recognize your current physiological state.

2. Tune in to the physical sensations accompanying your state.

3. Acknowledge your thoughts, emotions, and behaviors.

Your approach is personal and will vary depending on your circumstance. Avoid self-judgment and comparisons to others. Stay curious; there are no rigid rules of right or wrong.

Recognize Your Current Physiological State

Recognizing our physiological states as they shift throughout the day is invaluable because our states influence how we feel, think, and act. By stopping to check in with ourselves, we gain awareness of our current state and start to become familiar with what brought us there.

Our physiological states are transitory, shifting along the autonomic continuum as guided by our neuroception. Every state serves a purpose as an adaptation to our circumstances. It's important to recognize that not every moment will be in a ventral vagal state and that is not the goal. Instead, the goal is to be able to fluidly navigate among our states without getting stuck in a defensive state.

Observe your current state with compassion and acceptance. By cultivating awareness, we grow our resilience and we transform our ANS into an ally instead of our enemy.[2]

Tune In to the Physical Sensations
Accompanying Your State

How you feel in each of your physiological states can vary significantly. Paying attention to your physical sensations is a practical way to recognize your current state. For example, focus on your face and head. Do you notice any tension? Does a smile come naturally, or are you clenching your jaw? Are you particularly sensitive to sounds? Shift your focus to your chest. Is your heart racing? How would you describe your breathing? Does your body feel heavy or light and expansive?

Take a moment to simply notice and label these sensations without attaching a story to them based on past associations. This pause allows you to explore and become aware of how sensations can change depending on your circumstances.

Often, our feelings triggered by neuroception may not be directly linked to their actual sources. By focusing on the process of interoception without assuming a direct cause, we become open to investigating and understanding the triggers detected by our neuroception, which reliably influence our autonomic states of threat and safety. This helps us recognize our responses to specific stimuli and situations, reducing the influence of personal narratives that may falsely attribute intentional causality.

When we recognize the bodily sensations of our states, we can take appropriate actions to regulate our ANS and maintain equanimity. We can also better identify triggers for our states and learn how to manage those triggers. These capacities build with practice, just like any skill.

Acknowledge Your Thoughts, Emotions, and Behaviors

Being aware of and acknowledging our thought patterns, emotions, and behaviors provides valuable insight into how our nervous system reacts to the world around us. Through the lens of PVT, we can understand and soften our responses, leading to a more relaxed demeanor and reduced reactivity. This perspective also offers broader understanding that can enrich our relationships.

While the brain, especially the cortex, is often seen as the primary controller, it's important to recognize that our thought patterns, emotions, and behaviors are influenced by bodily sensations and our interpretations of them. By staying attuned to these sensations, we can better understand the origins of our thoughts, emotions, and behaviors.

Helpful Ways to Use the Regulation Toolbox

The Regulation Toolbox is offered to facilitate exploration of exercises and activities to enhance nervous system resilience. Organized by the primary autonomic states—connected ventral vagal, activated sympathetic, and shutdown dorsal vagal—the Regulation Toolbox offers a variety of activities and practices.

These activities complement SSP delivery and can be utilized before, during, and between client sessions. Prior to a session, both the provider and the client can engage in one or two activities to ensure readiness and accessibility during the session. Incorporating these activities during SSP sessions enhances the protocol's effectiveness. Between sessions, they assist in integrating changes and maintaining balance.

Because our nervous system is constantly responding to every moment we experience and adjusting to the stimuli around us, regulating it is an ongoing process that requires regular attention to maintain balance and well-being. Here are some ideas for making regular use of the Regulation Toolbox.

- **SELF-CARE:** Take a moment to check in on how you are feeling. Instead of powering through your day and to-do list, consider a short break to redirect your attention and give yourself some compassion and self-care.

- **PAUSE AND NOTICE:** After recognizing your current state, take a moment to become aware of how you are feeling in your body and what thought patterns and emotions you are experiencing.

- **EXPLORE:** Investigate the activities in the Regulation Toolbox that align with your current autonomic state. These self-care activities are designed to recalibrate your nervous system, promoting fluidity and reducing feelings of being stuck.

- **EXPERIMENT:** Try out each activity to determine which ones resonate best with you. Once you find a supportive activity, mark it for easy reference.

- **CUSTOMIZE:** Utilize the blank Regulation Toolbox in appendix 3 to personalize your own practices based on your unique individual nervous system states, sensations, thought patterns, emotions, behaviors, and preferences.

- **CONTINUE:** Keep returning to the Toolbox and other practices you use for nervous system balance and flexibility.

The Regulation Toolbox: Self-Directed Activities for Regulation by ANS State

Our well-being depends on our capacity to manage and balance our nervous system. In these toolboxes, you'll find numerous exercises and activities for autonomic regulation. Expanded descriptions are provided for activities that may not be self-evident.

VENTRAL VAGAL REGULATION TOOLBOX

Recognize Your Physiological State

Metaphor: We are in an inflatable boat—buoyant, easy to maneuver, and able to remain stable despite the wind and the waves.

Description: "We are floating."

Color: Green

Create Awareness of Your Physical Sensations

- Activated facial muscles—especially in the cheeks for smiling and around the eyes
- Warm/calm feeling in stomach
- Sense of body alignment and integration from head to toe
- Fluid movement
- Relaxed muscles
- Buoyant but grounded feelings
- Steady heart rate
- Elevated HRV
- Even breathing
- Positive energy
- Acute hearing
- Clear, prosodic voice

Acknowledge Your Thoughts, Emotions, and Behaviors

- Capable of compassion and understanding
- Calm and connected
- Aware and thinking clearly
- Present and "ready"
- Flexible
- Less concerned about the opinion of others and less negative in self-talk
- Mindful and embodied
- Able to access higher thinking processes and impulse control
- Creative, flexible, and playful
- Social
- Adaptable to change
- Open
- Bold—willing to take risks
- Able to think abundantly
- In awe

Activities for Regulation in a Ventral Vagal State

- Savor the feeling!
- Journal about what preceded this state so you can access it again more easily
- Connect and co-regulate with friends
- Appreciate the evenness of your breathing
- Stretch and welcome the freedom of movement

- Vocalize: hum, sigh, sing, whistle, laugh, play a wind instrument
- Move, walk, dance
- Meditate
- Listen to music that delights you
- Experience nature and what inspires you
- Engage in creative activities
- Activate your senses

SYMPATHETIC REGULATION TOOLBOX

Recognize Your Physiological State

Metaphor: We have tipped out of the boat and are actively struggling against the waves and currents.
Description: "We are flipping out."
Color: Red

Create Awareness of Your Physical Sensations

- Elevated heart rate
- Constricted breathing
- Lower HRV
- Anxious feelings
- Muscle tension
- Tight chest and throat
- Heightened arousal
- Restlessness
- Jitteriness
- Loss of integrated sense in body
- Disorganization
- Digestion difficulties
- Sleep difficulties
- Headaches
- Sweating
- Difficulty discerning speech; muted hearing
- Loud, tense, or shaky voice

Acknowledge Your Thoughts, Emotions, and Behaviors

- Anxious and insecure
- Focused on self, not others
- Hypervigilant
- Agitated
- Reactive (not responsive)
- Angry
- Thinking in black and white
- Unable to concentrate
- Experiencing racing thoughts
- Impulsive
- Irritable and confrontational
- Unable to think critically
- Overeating/overdrinking/overexercising
- Confrontational
- Fearful
- Sensitive to the perceived opinions of others
- Unable to connect with others

Activities for Regulation in a Sympathetic State

- Practice calming breathwork: extend or vocalize your exhale
- Practice Hand-on-Heart
- Vocalize: growl, sigh, hum, extend your phrases
- Practice Body sensing/scanning
- Notice areas of tension
- Practice progressive muscle relaxation
- Massage jaw and neck
- Move, shake, dance
- Practice Stanley Rosenberg's Basic Exercise
- Meditate
- Try something playful
- Connect and share with a friend
- Find humor
- Recall calming memories
- Feel comfort
- Practice the Valsalva Maneuver
- Experience nature and what calms you
- Practice Child's Pose
- Practice Box Breathing
- Practice Soothing Butterfly Hug
- Practice Simplified Self-Havening
- Practice Healing Head Hold
- Listen to calming music

DORSAL VAGAL REGULATION TOOLBOX

 Recognize Your Physiological State

Metaphor: We have sunk under the waves to seek protection and avoid the turbulence of the water's surface.

Description: "We are flopping down."

Color: Gray

Create Awareness of Your Physical Sensations

- Slow heart rate
- Shallow breathing
- Hollow stomach
- Slow movement, sedentariness
- Heavy body
- Hunched posture
- Low energy
- Dull, flat feelings
- Low gut motility
- Fatigue
- Oversleeping
- Dizzy
- Weak
- Nausea
- Muted hearing; difficulty discerning speech
- Monotone voice devoid of emotion or energy

Acknowledge Your Thoughts, Emotions, and Behaviors

- Disconnected
- Avoidant
- Numb
- On "auto pilot"
- Having difficulty remembering and concentrating
- Feeling flat emotionally
- Feeling negative
- Catastrophizing
- Ruminating
- Low on motivation
- Lacking creativity
- Overwhelmed
- Apathetic
- Hopeless
- Avoidant
- In a mental fog
- Having difficulty connecting with others

Activities for Regulation in a Dorsal Vagal State

- Be gentle with yourself
- Vocalize: groan, sigh, sing, hum
- Move, shift posture, stretch, wiggle fingers and toes, walk, rock, or sway
- Massage face, hands, and feet
- Practice activating breathwork, such as humming and bee breathing
- Experience nurturing sensations
- Take a shower or bath
- Wrap yourself in a blanket (even a weighted blanket)

- Massage your head
- Hug a pillow or a soft toy
- Recall a supportive connection with a friend; consider reaching out to them
- Experience nature and feel the sun, rain, or wind
- Listen to music you're drawn to
- Practice Stanley Rosenberg's Basic Exercise
- Practice Cat/Cow for awakening the body
- Practice Healing Head Hold
- Practice the Cross Crawl/Cross Over Shoulder Pull

Expanded Descriptions for Select Regulation Toolbox Activities

While many of the activities for regulation are straightforward and easy to understand, some benefit from further explanation. Following are more detailed descriptions of some of the regulation activities.

Breathwork

Breathwork provides a direct pathway to the nervous system and is a very efficient state shifter.[3] Moreover, our breath is always available to us. An extended exhale can promptly activate the vagal brake, slowing heart rate, while an intentional inhale can release the brake, infusing the system with energy. The heart naturally speeds up during inhalation and slows during exhalation. Activating breathwork prioritizes the inhale, while calming breathwork focuses on extending the exhale.

Donnalea Van Vleet Goeltz demonstrates breathing practices based on psychoeducational somatic intervention. A link is provided in the "Video Demonstration" section at the end of this chapter.

Stanley Rosenberg's Basic Exercise[4]

Repositioning the atlas (C1) and axis (C2) vertebrae in your upper spine increases mobility in the neck and spine and blood flow to the brainstem and can activate ventral vagal tone and access greater spontaneous social engagement. Lie on your back with your head cradled in your hands, interlacing your fingers and keeping your elbows wide. Without moving your head, slowly look as far to the right as possible using only your eyes. Hold briefly and then return your gaze to the ceiling. Repeat the eye movement to the left. Take your time and monitor your body's response, such as a yawn, sigh, or swallow, indicating relaxation. Be mindful when standing up afterward. To watch a video demonstration of the Basic Exercise performed by Arielle Schwartz, see the link in the "Video Demonstration" section at the end of this chapter.

Cat/Cow

A yoga sequence that involves moving between two poses, Cat/Cow helps with relaxation and ease. Begin in Tabletop Pose on your hands and knees with a flat back and, with an exhale, arch your spine upward and drop your head toward the floor for the "cat" position. Move through neutral and inhale into the "cow" position by pressing your chest forward and allowing your belly to sink. Your head and tailbone will be lifted toward the ceiling. Gently move between these two positions while shifting your breathing to increase circulation, spinal flexibility, and mobility.

Child's Pose

Child's Pose is a restorative yoga pose helpful for relaxation and rejuvenation. It releases tension in the back and shoulders and gently stretches the hips. Starting in Tabletop Pose, sit back on your heels and lower your torso forward, settling your chest between your thighs or as low as is comfortable. Spread your knees as wide as needed for you to breathe deeply. Extend your hands out in front of you, stretching through the arms. Relax and rest your forehead on the ground. You could also place a small ball under your forehead and gently roll from side to side for additional relief of nervous tension.

Box Breathing

Box Breathing is a rhythmic technique that has been used for thousands of years to engage the parasympathetic nervous system, aiding in anxiety relief and state shifting. It is a rhythmic breathing technique that involves four equal phases: inhale, hold, exhale, hold. You can do this practice anywhere and no one else needs to know what you are doing. Keep your eyes open or closed and inhale through your nose for a count of four, and then hold your breath for four. Exhale fully through your mouth or nose to the count of four, making sure all of the air is out of your lungs. After exhaling, pause and hold your breath for another count of four. Repeat the process for three to five minutes. You can use your attention to visualize tracing the sides of a box with your breath.

Hand-on-Heart

Hand-on-Heart is a self-soothing technique that is often used in meditation and stress reduction practices. This is an easy way to care for yourself with supportive touch. Like Box Breathing, you can do it anywhere discreetly. Touch (especially skin-to-skin contact) activates the parasympathetic nervous system and helps us to feel safe. Place one hand over your heart and put your other hand on top. Feel the gentle pressure and warmth of your hands. If comfortable, close your eyes and feel the rise and fall of your chest as you take slow, deep breaths. Use this exercise for self-compassion, calming, and centering.

The Valsalva Maneuver

The Valsalva Maneuver can act on the vagus nerve to slow your heart rate. It should not be used if you have heart disease, retinopathy, or an implanted eye lens. To do it, sit or lie down, close your mouth, and inhale deeply. Hold the breath in by also closing your windpipe in the throat. While keeping your airways closed (you may want to also pinch your nose shut), attempt to exhale forcefully as if trying to blow up a balloon. Wait at least a minute before repeating. Note that this maneuver should be cautiously implemented since it may also recruit dorsal vagal pathways and in combination with ventral pathways dramatically drop your heart rate and blood pressure sufficiently to cause dizziness or possibly fainting.

Soothing Butterfly Hug

This practice and the three that follow are courtesy of the Association for Comprehensive Energy Psychology's project, Resources for Resilience.[5]

Use the Soothing Butterfly Hug[6] when feeling emotional distress or anxiety to feel more heart centered, relaxed, and balanced. Cross your arms over your chest with one hand resting on each side of your upper chest. Alternate the movement of your hands gently tapping one side of the chest and then the other like the flapping wings of a butterfly. Breathe slowly and deeply until you feel calm and your thoughts have settled.

Simplified Self-Havening

Designed to calm and center the nervous system after a stressful or traumatic event, the Simplified Self-Havening[7] technique brings focus back to the body and the present moment. Cross your arms, each hand on the opposite shoulder. Slide your hands from both shoulders down to the elbows, with firm but gentle pressure. You can add humming and periodically rub your palms together.

Healing Head Hold

Use the Healing Head Hold[8] when feeling distressed, anxious, or unsettled. Place one hand across your forehead with the little finger across the eyebrows and the thumb up by the hairline. Lightly place the other hand at the base of the skull and hold the back of your head. Breathe. Hold this position until you feel calmer and can feel the pulse in your fingers. This should take three to five minutes. You can also hold a friend's head in the same way to shift their state and calm them.

The Cross Crawl/Crossover Shoulder Pull

The Crossover Shoulder Pull[9] can calm and rebalance the nervous system using bilateral stimulation. This can increase clarity and ability to focus. Draw your right hand from the top of your left shoulder to your right hip. Change hands and continue alternating.

Self-Regulating Activities for Children

The book *Howling with Huskies*[10] tells the story of how three Alaskan husky sled dogs teach sister and brother Galena and Kimmo about how to feel better when they experience difficult emotions. Written by Linda Chamberlain, PhD, MPH, a scientist and former dog musher, this book gives children self-regulating activities that can be done anytime and anywhere. Look for a link at the end of this chapter to a video demonstration of these and more activities for people of all ages provided by Dr. Chamberlain.

"Howling" or Quiet Sighing

Put one hand on your belly. Watch your belly fill like a balloon when you breathe in, then watch how it gets smaller as you let all the air out. If you like, you can take a breath in and make a long sound like a howling husky—"awoooooo"—as you let the air slowly out. Take a big breath in and let it out with a sound whenever you want to feel better. If you are in a place where you need to be quiet, you can breathe in and let it out with a whisper that only you can hear.

Holding Your Fingers

Look at your hand and name a feeling for each finger. Your thumb is sad. Your pointer is scared. Your middle finger is mad. Your ring finger is worried. And your little pinky finger is feeling bad. Choose a finger and a feeling you'd like to work with. You can use either hand. Now, wrap the fingers of your other hand around the finger you chose. Let's say you feel sad. Wrap your fingers around your thumb and while you do, think about feeling sad. Don't hold too tight. Take a few slow breaths and imagine you are breathing that feeling right out of the tip of your thumb. Try this for about a minute. If it's a big feeling, you can hold your finger longer. You can always hold your finger in your lap and no one will notice.

Shaking

When you feel excited and nervous at the same time, or you have too much energy inside you, you can shake it out! This will help you to feel calmer and more focused. Shake your arms and hands. Shake each leg, one at a time. Have fun and dance and shake your whole body!

Open Your Heart

Take a big breath in as you open your arms up to the sky. Then let the air out as you bring your hands to your heart. This can remind you to be kind to everyone.

Video Demonstrations of Activities for Regulation

Having an expert guide you through regulation activities offers valuable instruction and support. Access video guides from our polyvagal community at soundstrue.com/safe-and-sound-bonus.

- Jill Miller, C-IAYT, author of *Body by Breath* and *The Roll Model* and cofounder of tuneupfitness.com

   Jill demonstrates three zones to stimulate the vagus nerve and access areas of the body to aid in increased downregulation through breath and myofascial self-massage.

- Arielle Schwartz, PhD, drarielleschwartz.com

  Engage your vagus nerve naturally by exercising your eye muscles with Stanley Rosenberg's Basic Exercise. In his book *The Healing Power of the Vagus Nerve*, Rosenberg describes how moving your eyes can relax the occipital muscles, increasing blood flow to the brainstem and vagus nerve. Try eye exercises and neck stretches to experience these benefits firsthand.

- Amber Elizabeth Gray, PhD, ambergray.com

  The Yielding to Rise moving practice is an invitation to experience the dynamic range of neuro-physiological states—the literal dance of our vagal circuitry. Incorporating contemplative movement, somatic awareness, and more dynamic movement, this tiered practice will be shared in a way that is inclusive of all bodies and movement abilities.

- Jan Winhall, MSW, IPFOT, janwinhall.com

  The Felt Sense Polyvagal Grounding Practice is the foundational embodiment practice used in the Felt Sense Polyvagal Model. The practice teaches the two main embodied processes of interoception (felt sense) and neuroception (PVT).

- Betsy Polatin, MFA, SEP, AmSAT, humanual.com

  Two practices will be demonstrated. The Humanual Polyvagal Smile is an experiential exploration integrating the ventral vagal system with muscular, respiratory, and fascial systems, inviting awareness, discovery, and movement. The Exploration of Support considers the universal forces of gravity and antigravity and helps you connect to the ground and expand into your environment.

- Deb Dana, LCSW, rhythmofregulation.com

  Glimmers are micromoments of regulation that foster feelings of well-being. When we notice and name glimmers, we shape our system toward regulation. This practice helps you to see, stop, and appreciate glimmers as a way of shaping your nervous system toward regulation.

- Rebecca Bailey, PhD, LP, polyvagalequineinstitute.com

  The ability to be co-regulated and to co-regulate another is demonstrable across many human-animal interactions. Self-regulation and slowing down are prerequisites to connection, and for many people, this takes practice and the courage to connect. Horses are particularly aware of subtle communications of safety and bids for connection. In this brief video, you will see the communication in action between horse and human.

- Linda Chamberlain, PhD, MPH, GCFP, C-IAYT, drlindachamberlain.com

  Three simple tools for calming the body-brain and working with emotions will be demonstrated. Two of these tools are featured in *Howling with Huskies* along with other resources. These techniques can be used on the go and work for all ages.

- Donnalea Van Vleet Goeltz, PhD, continuummovement.com

  Breathing practices based on psychoeducational somatic intervention will be demonstrated. The approach is an educational and experiential learning process about one's nervous system using PVT and is currently being researched at University of Florida Health. Breathing techniques and movement are used to facilitate a change in physiological and psychological state.

Note: As with any holistic practice, it's advisable to consult with health-care professionals and use these regulating activities as complementary rather than alternative approaches to conventional medical care.

Part Two

Stories of Connection, Change, and Healing

The second part of this book offers real-life perspectives on the crucial role of the autonomic nervous system (ANS) in shaping our overall health, both physical and mental. Through case studies and stories, we explore the possibilities of the application of a polyvagal approach with Safe and Sound Protocol (SSP). As humans, we are inherently drawn to stories for deeper understanding. These narratives demonstrate the remarkable ability of our ANS to be retuned and our potential for change. Our goal is that, in addition to deepening your understanding of the ANS and polyvagal theory (PVT), these cases will inspire hope and optimism.

This book stems from decades of careful research, clinical experimentation, and the experiences of over 200,000 people who have undergone SSP. The case stories we present here are a tiny slice of this population, but they represent the vast possibilities of this polyvagal approach.

The cases are analyzed through the lens of PVT. While many other perspectives could also be applied, our emphasis remains on the impact of physiological states, social engagement, and the capacity of the ANS for change.

Conditions and Symptoms Addressed in the Case Studies

The cases that follow encompass a broad spectrum of conditions and a diverse range of scenarios. They include developmental trauma, PTSD, grief, shock, Parkinson's disease, flat facial affect, depressed SES, severe COVID, brain fog, fatigue, anxiety, depression, chronic pain, hypersensitivities, ear pain, hearing loss, perfectionism, sleep, suicidal ideation, suicide attempts, self-harm, academic stress, ADHD, auditory processing difficulty, hallucinations, dissociation, panic attacks, experience of war, attachment dynamics, selective mutism, social anxiety, gender dysphoria, speech disorders, addiction, and rapid onset dysregulation.

While SSP has indeed led to symptom reduction and has enhanced the lives of numerous clients, it's crucial to underscore that SSP should not be viewed as a cure for any physiological or psychological condition. Given its direct impact on the ANS and the wide-ranging influence of the ANS on the brain and body, SSP holds promise for improving numerous symptoms and conditions, often by promoting an autonomic state that facilitates the effectiveness of other treatments. However, while SSP can be greatly beneficial, it is not a panacea.

The Value of Case Studies and Stories

Case studies and stories play an important role in elucidating new therapeutic approaches like SSP. They offer real-world insights into the practical application of the therapy and provide tangible examples of its effects and outcomes. Through detailed accounts of individual experiences, case studies highlight the diverse circumstances, challenges, and transformations clients undergo with SSP. Additionally, the cases reveal the broader impact on the clients' social ecosystems, including their families, loved ones, schools, and communities.

While randomized control trials (RCTs) are essential for establishing the efficacy of interventions, they often overlook the richness of individual experiences. RCTs make a few observations about a lot of people, while case studies offer a lot of observations about a single person. And while each person participating in an RCT is unique, their individual stories, nuances, and intricacies may be overlooked in broader statistical analyses.

Recognizing the contributions of both evidence-based practice and practice-based evidence is important. While evidence-based practice provides a foundation rooted in established research findings, practice-based evidence offers invaluable insights gleaned from real-world clinical experience and observations.

By embracing the insights gained from case studies and stories, providers can adopt a more holistic and informed approach to SSP delivery, while clients can see their own experiences reflected in these narratives. These stories not only enhance our understanding of the therapy's effectiveness but also inspire ongoing exploration and refinement, laying the groundwork for future research and innovation in the field.

Case stories offer a window into the lives of others. The cases here tell the story of the nervous system. They reveal what happens when a person is trapped in a state of chronic defensiveness. We can see dysregulation and its far-reaching effects. Through these stories we learn to recognize the sensations, emotions, thoughts, and behaviors associated with different autonomic states and understand the experience of moving through the autonomic continuum and accessing greater balance. Each case provides valuable insights into effective strategies, empowering us to apply similar approaches in our own lives for meaningful change and growth.

Themes That Emerged from the Case Stories

The cases presented here cover a range of situations and conditions that may initially appear unrelated. However, when viewed through the lens of PVT, common themes emerge from both the providers' and clients' experiences with the SSP delivery process.

The Healing Power of PVT

In many cases, simply learning about PVT can initiate the healing process. Clients find PVT helpful because it explains how their body and brain react to stress and difficult experiences. They come to understand that their emotional and physiological reactions are adaptive and inherently geared toward self-preservation and growth. PVT elucidates why they feel certain emotions and how their body responds. This understanding is both validating and empowering as it assures them that achieving balance and flexibility in their nervous system is possible.

Navigating Back to a Ventral Vagal State

For many clients, accessing a ventral state of safety and connection seemed unattainable before SSP. However, during the process, it felt like discovering a lifeboat in a stormy sea. Being in a ventral vagal state provided relief and instilled hope for improvement.

As clients progress through SSP and repeatedly experience a ventral vagal state, they become more familiar with the sensations of safety and calmness in their body. This familiarity acts as a guidepost, making it easier to return to that state. While setbacks still occur, having this reference point reminds clients that a different, more positive experience is possible.

Unlocking Potential

Society loses immense potential when individuals are trapped in states of threat. The clients in these cases demonstrate how this potential can be unlocked and set free.

Harnessing Relationships for Change

Relationships and co-regulation are powerful stimulants for the vagus nerve. Particularly, an attuned connection with an SSP provider has proven to be a significant catalyst for growth and healing in many of the cases. Moreover, a recalibrated nervous system can enhance one's ability to engage authentically in relationships. Ultimately, relationships are the cornerstones of our health and contentment.

Safety Begets Safety

As clients lower their psychological defenses, their physiology often follows suit, initiating a positive upward spiral. By cultivating safety within the nervous system, clients in these cases reported reductions in both chronic psychological disturbances and physical issues. Given the reciprocal relationship between mental and physical conditions influenced by the ANS, improvements in one area often alleviate symptoms in the other.

Functional Disorders and Medically Unexplained Symptoms

The medical community frequently overlooks the neural regulation of our organs, leading many physical symptoms to be categorized as medically unexplained because their elusive origins remain unclear within traditional medical frameworks. These symptoms, which range from chronic pain and fatigue to gastrointestinal issues, autoimmune disorders, and voice and throat complaints, present substantial challenges for both patients and health-care providers. However, a deeper understanding of the interplay between neural regulation and bodily functions could offer novel insights into treating these conditions, as evidenced by some of these cases.

The Cyclic Defense Loop

Many of the clients experience the autonomic tendency known as the cyclic defense loop—a pattern of cycling between an activated sympathetic state and a shutdown dorsal vagal state. This pattern traps them in a vicious downward spiral. However, the abundant safety provided by SSP and the support of the provider offer a way out of this cycle.

Foundational Safety

Was this person's need for safety met during early development? This question was pivotal in every case. Early experiences of safety significantly increase the likelihood of connecting with and trusting one's provider. For those who lacked early experiences of love and safety, SSP has supported their capacity for self-regulation and, eventually, connection and co-regulation. Repetition of SSP sessions or SSP boosters may offer additional support for individuals with developmental trauma.

Individualized Delivery of SSP

The cases illustrate a diverse range of delivery approaches. Recognizing that every nervous system, situation, and day is unique, there is no one-size-fits-all approach to SSP delivery.

Our Capacity for Change

Our nervous system patterns are shaped by our life experiences and our habits. The opposite is also true: our habits and actions can change our nervous system patterns. SSP serves as a catalyst for experiencing life in a new way and establishing new patterns for the clients in these cases.

A Guide to the Case Study Format

Each case is structured with a standardized format for consistency, context, and ease of navigation. The following are the key sections of each case study:

- Case overview: Provides essential details about the SSP provider, the client, assessments used, and the client's autonomic tendency.

- Client description: A detailed profile of the client, including background information, motivation for seeking SSP, prominent symptoms, and therapeutic goals.

- SSP delivery method: Description of how SSP was delivered, including psychoeducation, session structure, titration process, playlist and pathways used, and any concurrent modalities.

- Summary of provider's observations about the client's response to SSP: Narrates changes observed by the provider, including client feedback and reflections during the delivery process.

- Assessments: Summarizes assessment results (when utilized). Descriptions of the assessments are provided in appendix 1.

- Summary of client's reflections on their response to SSP: The client's perspective on their SSP experience, including input from family members or friends if applicable. If the client is a child, the reflections are provided by their parent(s).

- Case analysis with Dr. Porges: Following the completion of each case write-up, a comprehensive discussion involving Dr. Porges, Karen Onderko, and the SSP provider and their client ensued. Insights gleaned from this dialogue, combined with the case content, were utilized to provide a thorough analysis of each case from a polyvagal perspective.

- Implications for daily life: At the end of each case study, a brief reflection explores how the lessons learned from the client's experience can be applied in personal life.

Key polyvagal insights vividly demonstrate PVT in action. Rather than including these insights in a separate section in each case study, we highlight pivotal moments throughout each case where these polyvagal insights are evident, with footnotes provided to contextualize these moments. The polyvagal insights are described in appendix 4 for reference.

How the Cases Were Selected

Assembling the cases for this book was much like piecing together a complex jigsaw puzzle. Each piece was carefully selected to create a comprehensive and balanced representation of SSP's impact across various contexts.

Our goal was to ensure that the cases presented in part 2 reflect the wide spectrum of diversity among providers, including their various disciplines and modalities. We also aimed to capture a broad range of clients, along with their unique characteristics and symptoms.

Moreover, we wanted to showcase the different approaches to SSP delivery and the breadth of outcomes achieved. Rather than focusing on the most dramatic or surprising results, we aimed to illustrate the kinds of outcomes that are commonly observed when SSP is delivered with genuine connection and attunement. By doing so, we hope to offer readers a deeper understanding of how clinicians are effectively integrating SSP into their practice with clients.

In addition, we included cases where the results were unexpected to emphasize that even unanticipated responses can be valuable and worked with effectively. These cases demonstrate the flexibility and adaptability of SSP delivery, showing that every outcome, whether anticipated or not, holds potential for growth and healing.

Provider and Client Backgrounds

The providers featured in these cases represent a diverse cross section of the overall provider community. They span 10 clinical disciplines and employ 20 different modalities in their practices. While most providers are from the US, others hail from four other countries. The provider group includes 1 male provider and 12 female providers.

Among the clients, six are from countries outside the US. The group includes three men, six women, and six children (three girls and three boys), with three identifying as LGBTQIA+. Overall, four races and eight ethnicities are represented in the cases.

Privacy and Accuracy

Every participant in the case studies was offered the option of anonymity through the use of pseudonyms and/or slight alterations to specific locations or unique circumstances. Ultimately, 9 of the 13 cases in this book use pseudonyms, which are clearly indicated in the case overview summaries.

Each case was meticulously developed through close collaboration among the authors, the SSP provider, and the client to ensure accuracy and authenticity. Every case underwent multiple readings and thorough scrutiny, with each participant's approval obtained before the case was included in the book. This rigorous approach was designed to uphold the integrity of the work and honor the individuals involved in the case studies.

An Ongoing Conversation

We hope for this book to be the start of a conversation that will continue to unfold over time. Just as the impact of SSP on a client will continue to evolve and expand over time, our understanding of best practices and the mechanisms involved will inevitably grow and develop. We encourage you, whether as clinicians or clients, to reflect on your own experiences and outcomes. This may lead to new insights and innovative approaches.

By recognizing and clarifying the diverse responses to SSP, a deeper appreciation of the role and wide-ranging effects of the ANS may result. When the core impact of the ANS is fully grasped, we can give it the respect and support it deserves as the source of physiological and psychological health. This is optimistic for the future of SSP and the many ways it can be applied in our lives.

When the nervous system is retuned toward safety, abundant wellness becomes attainable. When clients are transitioning out of a defensive state, they become open to health, change, and growth. They report increased sociability, enhanced cognitive abilities, improved auditory processing and listening acuity, reduced hypersensitivities, better emotional regulation, and an overall sense of well-being. These transformative effects are detailed in the following chapters.

Chapter 5

From Rapid Onset Dysregulation to Restoration

Case Overview

SSP PROVIDER: Tracy Murnan Stackhouse, MA, OTR/L, pediatric occupational therapist, executive director, director of programs, and cofounder of Developmental FX. Website: developmentalfx.org

CLINICAL DISCIPLINE: Occupational therapy

OTHER THERAPEUTIC MODALITIES AND EXPERTISE: Sensory integration, DIR/Floortime, neurodevelopmental treatment, Treatment and Education of Autistic and Related Communication Handicapped Children, Early Start Denver Model, craniosacral therapy and myofascial release, and Theraplay

CLIENT: Catie (a pseudonym) is a six-year-old girl in kindergarten. Prior to coming down with a virus, she was a playful, outgoing little girl with many friends. Following a brief virus, she was suddenly struggling with significant anxiety and disruption to her social and emotional functioning with impacts across all areas of functioning.

FEATURES/SYMPTOMS: Sudden onset of anxiety and OCD-like behavior following a brief virus. Primary concerns were separation anxiety, extreme dysregulation, sensory defensiveness, flat affect, restricted food choices, poor sleep, reduced social engagement, and frequent self-soothing techniques, including genital stimulation.

AUTONOMIC TENDENCY: Prior to the virus and onset of difficulties, Catie was in a ventral vagal state most of the time. At the onset of treatment, she mostly oscillated between sympathetic and dorsal states (the cyclic defense loop) with a constant sense of unease and fear.

ASSESSMENTS: Parent interview, clinical observation, and the Short Sensory Profile were used in the intake process, but no formal post-SSP assessments were utilized.

Client Description

Catie, a kindergarten-aged girl, lived with her parents (mom and dad) and an older brother. Prior to the challenges outlined here, she had started kindergarten just two months earlier at the school where her mother was an administrator. She was a typically developing, healthy, and joyful child with a wide circle of friends. Catie exuded a delightful zest for play and excelled in swimming and loved doing tumbling/gymnastics at home. Her interactive style was charming, often delighting in tricking familiar adults. She relished playing with her peers, eagerly engaged in academic activities and art projects, and had a keen interest in being a classroom helper.

Following a mild virus, Catie experienced the sudden onset of anxiety and OCD-like behavior, which significantly disrupted her daily life functioning and school attendance. This prompted her parents to seek medical and therapeutic support. Upon referral to Tracy for occupational therapy, Catie presented with several challenges. The primary concerns were anxiety and extreme dysregulation, compounded by sensory defensiveness that limited her clothing choices and increased discomfort in various situations. She exhibited heightened anxiety, persistent unnamable fears, and a flattened affect, movement, and energy. Notably, she displayed intense attention on handwashing and wiping after using the toilet, along with frequent trips to the bathroom and increased time there, particularly on the toilet. Additionally, her food choices became restricted, and her eating and sleeping patterns deteriorated in quality and quantity.

Also troubling for her parents was her use of self-soothing techniques that included genital stimulation for many hours each day. School attendance became increasingly difficult, and her relationships with peers and adults suffered. Catie strongly preferred close physical proximity to her mother, even for sleep, with a reduced willingness for other adults to offer her support or comfort. Recognizing the severity of Catie's symptoms, her parents sought medical guidance and therapeutic support from a mental health counselor and pediatrician, in addition to occupational therapy with Tracy.

Tracy's occupational therapy intake evaluation with the Short Sensory Profile revealed increased primitive postural reflexes and startle responses in Catie. She had a reduction in play activity and had regressed in her fine motor skills, using a palmar grasp, which uses the entire palm and fingers to secure an object—a pattern seen in newborns—instead of the more refined dynamic grasp she had previously used. Catie's sudden onset of sensory defensiveness reduced her range of food choices and clothing items (to primarily one pair of pants). She was less able to engage in and attend to academic tasks and her problem-solving ability was reduced. This led to emotional dysregulation and poor adaptive functioning.

Catie was evaluated by her primary care provider, who referred her to specialists in neurology and psychiatry. Catie's mom also reached out to personal contacts in immunology and neurology to gather more information. Catie's initial anxiety was so intense that she was given hydroxyzine hydrochloride to assist with sleep and temporary anxiety support. After an MRI and EEG, no focal neurological findings were reported, though the soft signs reported in the OT evaluation were noted. While a virus was the precipitating factor, a formal diagnosis of PANS (Pediatric Acute-Onset Neuropsychiatric Syndrome) or PANDAS (pediatric autoimmune neuropsychiatric disorders associated with streptococcal infections) was not officially given, though it was speculated and remains within the range of possible clinical considerations.

SSP Delivery Method

Catie was dysregulated most of each day. She alternated between being angry and irritable to crying and shutting down. She needed to be close to her mother and also used self-soothing strategies. SSP within the context of OT intervention was selected to address the autonomic dysregulation that accounted for most of her presenting problems.

An initial three-week intensive intervention burst was suggested to address the changes in her functioning. Sessions were scheduled four to five times per week. Catie's treatment plan emphasized the importance of considering Catie's unique sensory needs and preferences in the context of her environmental, personal, and social contexts. The goals were to reduce sensory defensiveness, restore a calm ventral vagal state, develop a felt sense of safety, improve interoceptive awareness, and increase overall coping skills in support of maintaining state regulation across environments and typical daily challenges that might trigger dysregulation. Above all, warm connection, predictability, and safety were prioritized in every step of the process.

SSP Core was delivered in person at the clinic over the course of three weeks, comprising a total of 15 sessions with five hours dedicated to listening. From the very first session, which consisted of a seven-minute listening segment, a noticeable calming effect was observed in Catie, with a reduction in agitation and worry. Building upon this positive response, subsequent sessions extended the listening time, with Catie actively requesting more listening. Additional elements such as movement activities, like exploring a ramp and swinging in a Lycra hammock, were interspersed with listening segments, enhancing Catie's engagement and comfort.

To create a cozy and inviting environment for listening, a pile of soft pillows was arranged, leading to the term "cuddle puddle" as Catie, her mother, and Tracy settled in together. Percy, the weighted plush animal, a penguin game, and craft time provided continuity and comfort throughout the sessions. As the week progressed, Catie's enthusiasm for therapy grew, evident in her eagerness to attend sessions and her proactive involvement in setting up the cuddle puddle and selecting therapeutic tools.

Listening sessions increased in duration in the first week, reaching 30 minutes per session by the third day before taking a break for the weekend. During the subsequent week, the 30-minute sessions in the clinic were complemented by 30-minute sessions at home, with Mom as the co-regulator. Catie's enthusiasm and active participation in therapy grew with each visit, reflecting her increasing comfort and engagement with the therapeutic process. Following the intensive phase of therapy, selected sessions of SSP Core (Hours 3 and 4) and SSP Balance were integrated into a home program spanning three additional months, totaling seven hours of listening.

During this extended phase, monthly sessions with Tracy were scheduled to monitor the stability of Catie's symptoms and to maintain the therapeutic connection she valued. It was important to gradually reduce the frequency of sessions to allow Catie to develop trust in other co-regulatory partners while ensuring continued support for her ongoing developmental needs. Concurrently, efforts were made to consolidate active self-regulation skills and reinforce psychoeducation both at home and school.

Summary of Provider's Observations about the Client's Response to SSP

When Catie's mother first contacted Tracy, the overwhelming sense of concern she conveyed about her daughter's well-being struck Tracy deeply. The swift progression from the onset of the virus to the significant decline in Catie's daily functioning was difficult to comprehend.

As some family members had a history of struggles with anxiety, there was some understanding of the emotional challenges Catie was facing, but the disappearance of her happiness and onset of coping attempts that were intensely driven and difficult to understand was truly distressing. It left her mother and father grappling with grief, overwhelming worry, and a profound sense of hopelessness.

Adding to the family's distress was the lack of clarity regarding the situation—no identified cause, no clear path forward, and conflicting advice from medical professionals, some of which involved costly and invasive testing procedures. The results had all come back to the suggestion that this was a mental health event to be resolved with medication and behavioral support. Despite the suggestions of mental health interventions, this didn't resonate with the family's experience.

Tracy viewed the situation through the lens of PVT. While diagnosing the cause of Catie's difficulties was beyond her scope, the constellation of symptoms suggested dysregulation of her ANS. Whether this dysregulation stemmed directly from the virus or its aftermath, it was evident that addressing her regulatory system was imperative.

In the initial sessions, Catie was timid, often hiding behind her mother, reminiscent of a toddler in a new social setting. Despite her desire to engage and connect, she seemed constrained by internal barriers. This was a poignant reality for her mother, who witnessed the stark contrast from Catie's previous vibrant self. As her mother courageously held space for these changes, she grappled with her own fears and worries about Catie's future well-being. Acknowledging and validating both Catie's and her mother's fears, while fostering a sense of safety, became paramount in the sessions.

As treatment progressed, a gradual return to regulation was marked by Catie's increasing access to the calmer and more engaging ventral vagal state—much to the relief of both her and her mother. Throughout the course of therapy, there were moments that resonated deeply, akin to "falling in love," evoking a profound sense of connectedness that often moved Catie's mother to silent tears as she witnessed her child's reemergence.

Each session in the clinic included periods of active listening to the next segment of SSP, often facilitated in the "cuddle puddle" space. They incorporated the penguin game, which seamlessly integrated opportunities for shared social touch—a nurturing aspect that Catie

---

* Polyvagal Insight 4: The Power of Social Connection and Co-Regulation

had avoided during the most challenging times of her journey. She began to embrace moments of quiet exchange, such as using lotion to soften their hands for holding the penguins or exchanging eggs, symbolizing care and connection. Each session included collaborative problem-solving activities centered on assisting the penguins, fostering a sense of prosocial connectedness that played a crucial role in strengthening Catie's ventral state.

Furthermore, they engaged in motor exploration activities with progressively increasing challenges, addressing Catie's emerging postural motor difficulties and reigniting her passion for gymnastics. Craft activities were utilized to target fine motor skills while grounding shared experiences during the listening portions of the session. Cultivating access and awareness of the ventral state of regulation was the primary goal. As therapy progressed, Catie began to radiate her inner sparkle; to spend time with her was to experience her joyful light.

Psychoeducation played a pivotal role in Catie's treatment, and SSP served as the primary catalyst for change. Through telehealth, psychoeducation sessions were conducted with Catie's parents, as well as with her school team, to establish a shared understanding of the regulation model drawn from PVT. This model was simplified and tailored for Catie, fostering her curiosity and engagement with concepts such as interoceptive awareness, active self-regulation, and self-compassion.

As therapy continued, Catie explored more strategies for use at home and school, enhancing her self-regulation and resilience. Fostering a shared understanding among Catie, her family, and her school team created a supportive environment for her development and well-being.

The goal to proportionally replace her self-soothing and toileting-focused actions with states of ventral regulation and alternate body-based coping skills was realized. SSP was used throughout the course of the intensive direct treatment and then titrated to completion. The other regulation strategies were solidified as a part of daily life at home and school and continued past the point of discharge from therapy.

In the follow-up period, Catie experienced a mild regression in her handwashing and toileting routines due to a norovirus illness. While much less intense, there was a return of self-soothing self-touch and an increased need for proximity with her mom. Her mother worried they were returning to a period of dysregulation. But with a few added SSP sessions and reinforcement of the other self-regulation and interoceptive supports, it resolved and Catie returned to doing well. This event underscored the importance of maintaining a lifestyle that supports Catie's well-being as essential.

Summary of the Parent's Reflections on Their Child's Response to SSP

Catie's mom described how Catie went to bed on a Sunday night—"her happy, joyful, and spunky self"—and woke up on Monday with "extreme separation anxiety and OCD behaviors." As the days went on, Catie would go from yelling, screaming, hitting, and not wanting to get dressed in the morning to crying in a fetal position, like a one-and-a-half-year-old, exhausted and frustrated. This would happen again at night. During the day, she experienced separation anxiety. Catie's parents were confused, frustrated, and frightened. They frantically searched for connections to doctors, therapists, or anyone in their community who could help.

The teachers and staff rallied around Catie and her family, providing tremendous support and understanding. They could see that Catie needed help—and fast. One of her teachers said, "Catie is gone and we need to get her back." Her teachers worked hard to make sure Catie felt safe, but they acknowledged that there was "no road map" to follow. Still, they found ways to normalize Catie's situation for the other children and support Catie in special and caring ways.

Despite how "amazing" her teachers were, it was difficult to get Catie to school, and when she was there, she cried and spent about two hours of each day in the bathroom. Catie's mom walked her from her office to Catie's classroom each morning. They would spend 20 minutes in the bathroom and when they finally entered the classroom, Catie needed to be "peeled off" of her.

By the time Catie's parents reached out to Tracy, Catie had had symptoms for six and a half weeks. Tracy was the first medical professional who truly listened to their concerns and gave some hope with a treatment plan. Many of the other professionals they had seen were unfamiliar with this type of reaction to a virus and did not know much about PANDAS or PANS. The parents were relieved to find someone who understood that this was more than a mental health issue.

By the end of the first session with Tracy, it was clear that this was a promising path for Catie, and her parents felt optimistic about the potential benefits. Before leaving that day, they scheduled every available appointment with Tracy and saw her almost every weekday for the next three weeks. Tracy's presence was healing, providing not only comfort for Catie but also reassurance for her mom, who felt fully supported throughout the process. Catie's small circle of trust easily widened to include Tracy. And there was never a session where Catie's mom did not cry tears of relief.

Catie did some listening at home with mom and, while they did notice changes, it was not the same as when Tracy was with them. Catie's responses were that much better with Tracy. Catie became increasingly more present in her body and was clearly more regulated. Now, when she walked into the clinic, her posture changed from previously being a bit stooped as she "guarded her core" to "walking tall with her shoulders back." This change began to extend to all areas of her life.[*]

Catie "came back little by little." Her mom described that anyone paying attention to their situation noticed this too. Catie tapered off her self-soothing and reliance on rituals. She also started falling asleep more easily. Within six months, Catie confidently walked to her classroom with her brother. She reestablished her relationships and had good friends again. She felt "important" and appreciated by other people.

Catie hasn't fully returned to her former self, but her joyful nature is gradually returning. "We see her more and more," the family described. But viruses affect Catie uniquely, and Tracy wisely cautioned that this

---

[*] Polyvagal Insight 7: The ANS Can Be Retuned to Prioritize Connection and Well-Being

process could take multiple years. When she gets sick, some of her dys-regulated behaviors return. Nevertheless, Mom notes that "Catie's worst days now were her best days then."

Catie was still very sensitive and needed lots of hugs and soothing pressure. Following the initial virus, she frequently was irritable and operated autonomously. But her OCD behaviors ceased and only briefly resurfaced during illness. Instead, sickness tended to evoke intense emotions and heightened separation anxiety in Catie. Tracy's support and SSP provided background reassurance during those times. If Catie got sick again, her mom knew where to find supportive resources. She had confidence that spending time with Tracy and listening to more SSP would help Catie to recover quickly.

Case Analysis with Dr. Porges

Catie's ANS mounted a quick and intense response to the virus she was exposed to. Overnight, her physiology shifted into a heightened defensive mode, compromising her abilities to both self-regulate to calm herself and co-regulate to be soothed through interactions with others.[*] This unexpected array of defensiveness rendered her nearly unrecognizable to her parents.

Virus Triggers Defensive Response

Although her sickness resolved within days, Catie's nervous system was reluctant to relinquish its defenses. It appeared that it was locked in a state of defense and extreme coping attempts, although her bodily reactions had effectively neutralized the pathogen. It was as if her nervous system organized the mechanisms to overcome the illness but was not informed through normal neural feedback pathways that the defensive strategies could be discontinued.

---

[*] Polyvagal Insight 2: Autonomic States Bias Our Feelings, Thoughts, and Behaviors

Defensive Nervous System Responses
Trigger Behavioral Reactions

The highly defensive response of Catie's ANS compromised her access to the neural circuits necessary to calm and co-regulate via the SES. In the absence of a functional SES with access to the calming ventral vagal pathways, her sympathetic and dorsal vagal states took over. In a way, the depressed SES provided the "neural permission" for unopposed sympathetic excitation with the associated hypersensitivities that trigger and maintain defensiveness. However, sympathetic activation is metabolically costly and cannot be maintained. Thus, her behavioral exhaustion led to an autonomic rebound of immobilization through dorsal vagal pathways, further contributing to her being locked in a state of autonomic dysregulation.

The sympathetic signs were observed in her behavior as tactile defensiveness (restricting her to a single pair of pants), auditory hypersensitivity (reacting to sounds like toilet flushing and certain voices), physiological responses (muscle tension, facial flushing, and having gastrointestinal issues), and selective eating.

The sensation of dysregulation in her body was discomforting, making emotional regulation and connection challenging. She sought solace and safety from her mother and struggled to cope when apart from her. Frequently inconsolable, she discovered self-soothing through self-touch as a means to alleviate her distress. This may have been an unconscious strategy to "protect" Catie's nervous system from dropping deeper into dorsal vagal regulation.

Auditory Sensitivity

Socially, Catie was having difficulty finding comfort in relationships. She began avoiding interactions with her father and her grandfather and refraining from visiting her grandparent's house—a place she previously cherished. Her avoidance of the important male figures in her life may have stemmed from her increased auditory sensitivity and her defensive state, which amplified the low frequencies of their voices and biased her neuroception to detect further threat.*

It is important to note that our nervous system, similar to other mammals, is wired with a bias toward detecting low-frequency vocalizations as predator signals. When in a state of threat, according to PVT, middle ear muscle tone is reduced, amplifying the loudness of low-frequency voices such as those typically spoken by fathers, who generally speak in a lower frequency band compared to mothers. Within the SSP provider community, there have been several reports of children expressing fearful reactions to male voices. The potency of this trigger has also been reported to disappear following SSP, which can be hypothetically explained by the reengagement of the middle ear muscles that dampen the loudness of voices expressed in lower frequencies.

Catie's own voice also changed in response to her state, shifting to a higher frequency expressed as "baby talk." The quality of one's voice reflects their autonomic state. In a defensive state, the voice may lose its rhythm and prosody and shift to lower or higher frequencies.†

Gastrointestinal Issues

Gastrointestinal issues can serve as another indicator of one's autonomic state. For instance, constipation typically signals a sympathetic dominance, while loose bowels suggest a dorsal vagal response. Catie's selective eating, toileting difficulties, and hyperfocus on wiping reflected her fluctuating states. As she traversed through the cyclic defense loop, her variations of defensiveness could be discerned through her bowel movements. Recently, when she encountered another virus, she experienced stomach pain followed by loose bowels. This dorsal vagal reaction aligns with a neuroception of the virus as a life-threatening event.

Catie's ANS appears to be adapting, as evidenced by her ability to rebound from illness and widespread dysregulation. Going forward, her stomach condition and excretions can serve as vital clues and early indicators of dysregulation.

---

* Polyvagal Insight 6: Autonomic State, Vocal Intonation, and Middle Ear Muscle Regulation Mutually Influence Each Other

† Polyvagal Insight 5: Autonomic State Impacts Social Cues

The ANS and the Brain-Body Connection

While her constellation of symptoms confounded many doctors, PVT suggests they were a reflection of an ANS that had shifted into a state of protection and out of one of connection and homeostasis.* Catie's symptoms were a representation of her nervous system's attempt to deal with the threat. The threat was a virus, but other experiences such as a physical injury, bullying, emotional abuse, or other traumas may have initiated similar defensive responses. The disruption Catie experienced was very real despite the fact that no antibodies to strep were detected and a diagnosis could not be confirmed by the multiple tests that were administered.

Without a clear understanding of the central regulatory nature of the ANS, the medical professionals involved in her care presumed that her experience was due to a mental health event. While this did not resonate with anyone in Catie's life, it was disruptive to everyone. Her parents, especially, were confused and concerned, and their own nervous systems became dysregulated, likely further deepening Catie's pattern of oscillating between activated sympathetic and shutdown dorsal states. Likewise, her state was affecting theirs too, as autonomic states are contagious.

Importantly, Catie's presentation suggested many namable mental health conditions, but none of these would have addressed the root issue as residing in autonomic dysregulation. Catie's story emphasizes the key role the ANS has in our wellness and mental health needs.

Moreover, the inability to detect the root cause of her symptoms could have hindered her access to adequate support and treatment, placing Catie at further risk. While her symptoms resembled those of PANS, once it was clear that she did not require antibiotics, the priority became to ensure she received suitable treatment for her symptoms of ANS dysregulation.

Cues of Safety Retune the ANS Toward Homeostasis

Tracy's ability to see through Catie's symptoms to her nervous system and her confidence that she had tools to help resolve them was the beginning of Catie's recovery. Tracy became a through line of safety, providing

---

* Polyvagal Insight 8: The ANS Is at the Core of Our Physical and Mental Wellness

a safe haven for Catie and her family. She understood that her first role was to provide abundant cues of safety to the whole family. Catie's mom too was quite instrumental in this same way. Both Tracy and Catie's mom used regulation, reassurance, and rituals to offer a supportive environment for healing. This helped SSP to do its job.[*]

Regulation

Tracy provided psychoeducation to Catie and the family about how her nervous system was trying to protect her and how SSP could improve her regulation, sociality, and symptoms of hypersensitivity. This context provided a sense of relief.

She also helped Catie discover activities, such as breathing exercises, that would help her feel calmer. Playing a kazoo was suggested as a fun and easy way to extend her exhale, which is calming. The family also has access to SSP Balance to provide an in-the-moment state shifter. These alternate ways to regulate herself began to replace her self-soothing.

Reassurance

The combined warmth and tenderness shown by Tracy, Catie's parents, brother, and extended family, and her teachers—evident in their attentive care and comforting presence—provided Catie with a profound sense of love and security. The cuddle puddle, games, and sleeping with her mother all reassured Catie and her nervous system that she was loved and would not be judged or rejected due to her behaviors.

Rituals

Catie knew right where to go first when she arrived at Tracy's clinic: to the cuddle puddle pillow pile. Before their morning routine of walking to her classroom, Mom and Catie drew small hearts on their hands and "filled up their hearts" by touching them together. They would say to each other, "You are safe and you are loved" over and over again. Her teachers also repeated that mantra to her. And, each morning, when they walked into the classroom, her teachers would give Catie a big hug with

---

* Polyvagal Insight 1: Autonomic State Functions as an Intervening Variable

pressure and walk her over to the "Question of the Day" board and help her fill it out. They would sit with her until her body calmed.

In the midst of the sudden upheaval in her life, these rituals provided the sense of predictability and safety that Catie was desperate for. The predictability of rituals and daily routines were comforting and provided a form of safety, or "neural expectancy," when everything else was uncertain.

These approaches, together with SSP and Tracy's clarity and support, set Catie on a path toward recovery and a return to her former self after enduring this challenging episode in her life.

Implications for Daily Life

Illness and other disruptors can cause dysregulation of the ANS, typically as an adaptive and protective response. Recognizing this mechanism can help ease concerns about symptoms, even when the dysregulation seems severe. Catie's recovery underscores a critical lesson: while context and developmental history may contribute to symptoms, through a polyvagal lens, the symptoms and challenges are understood as the consequences of shifts in ANS state, not as a mental health crisis or a permanent retuning of the nervous system.

Furthermore, the role of supportive caregivers is crucial in this context. Their ability to regulate, reassure, and maintain consistent rituals provides essential support for those in their care. The involvement of parents, teachers, and therapists who offer their empathy and connectedness plays a vital role in the healing process. Their presence and understanding not only aid in navigating the dysregulation but also help in restoring balance and promoting overall well-being.

Chapter 6

Hannah Rediscovers Her Voice and Vitality

Case Overview

> **SSP PROVIDER:** Heleen Grooten, SLP, SEP. Website: heleengrooten.nl/English
>
> **CLINICAL DISCIPLINE:** Speech therapist for over 40 years focusing on breathing and voice therapies with a special interest in unexplained somatic complaints and features related to trauma and dysregulation of the ANS
>
> **OTHER THERAPEUTIC MODALITIES AND EXPERTISE:** Somatic Experiencing, mindfulness, voice/breathing therapy, and Systemic Constellations
>
> **CLIENT:** Hannah (a pseudonym), a mental health professional in her 50s in the Eastern Netherlands, had been in therapy for years to address the effects of multiple childhood traumas. Five years after the death of her longtime partner, she still experienced a loss of joy and zest for life.
>
> **FEATURES/SYMPTOMS:** Grief, chronic pain, complex trauma, muscle tension, globus pharyngeus (a sensation of a lump or foreign object in the throat, despite there being no physical obstruction), vocal impairment, and jaw clenching
>
> **AUTONOMIC TENDENCY:** Dorsal vagal shutdown
>
> **ASSESSMENTS:** Beyond Heleen's standard intake process and measures, no formal assessments were utilized.

Client Description

Hannah was a mental health professional with multiple adverse childhood experiences and a diagnosis of complex trauma. Long-term psychotherapy had been supportive to her and improved her life. She had developed more secure relationships and experienced less suffering from intrusive memories.

Five years before meeting Heleen, she witnessed the violent death of her partner with whom she had lived for more than 25 years. Both her attachment issues and PTSD symptoms flared up again.

Her loss was still traumatic for her. She was living alone, withdrawn from friends and family, and was easily triggered. She lacked the interest and energy to maintain a healthy life balance and had lost her vitality and inner spark.

Physically she had several complaints. At times, her heart lost its usual rhythm and began to beat irregularly and faster than normal. This made her feel restless and tired. Pain in her groin prevented her from walking or otherwise being physically active for more than 20 minutes. She had tight shoulders and tension in her neck and upper back. Last, she experienced clenching of her jaw and a "closed" feeling in her throat and larynx, sometimes more like a lump in her throat, other times more like suffocating (globus pharyngeus). Her voice was pinched and more constricted than usual. As a mental health clinician, she knew that her emotional and physical symptoms were intertwined with her stress and trauma history.

Hannah had learned about SSP from a workshop Heleen had given on PVT and SSP. Hannah was intrigued that such a simple intervention could be so effective, but she was also wary that if SSP could bypass conscious control to change one's physiology, it might evoke a lot of painful emotions and memories. At the same time, she was curious and wanted to try it out as soon as she could. Her first chance to have enough time and space for whatever might emerge was the upcoming anniversary of her partner's death for which she had already arranged to take two weeks off from work. This was historically a difficult time of year for her, when she would find that her attention was poor, making her prone to mistakes. She trusted Heleen's judgment and ability to co-regulate with her, as well as her own ability to take care of herself. She notified her psycho-therapist of her plan.

She was hoping to regain physical health and mental stability. Her true wish, although she was skeptical, was the possibility of rediscovering her inner fire—to be able to live with passion again.

SSP Delivery Method

SSP Core was delivered to Hannah in nine sessions, over 17 days, for 20–60 minutes per session.

The general structure of each session was to first spend time getting reacquainted and review the sensations and experiences that Hannah had had since the previous session. Then Heleen and Hannah discussed PVT and the impact of Hannah's physiological state on her sensations, emotions, thoughts, and behaviors. In each session, Heleen made sure the room was set up in a way that put Hannah at ease and checked with her to see if anything was needed (coffee, tea, a pillow or blanket, shoes on or off), all to ensure that Hannah felt as comfortable as possible.

Heleen was alongside Hannah during all of the listening sessions. She was attentive to Hannah's state and paid close attention to her body movements, facial expressions, and general reactions to the music. Heleen was mindful of Hannah's comfort level with eye contact and shifted her gaze toward the window periodically.

Hannah was able to be explicit about her bodily state as it shifted while listening to SSP. She reported a variety of bodily sensations including tightness in her stomach, a fluttering heart rate, dizziness, tension in her throat and jaw, movement in her larynx, deeper breathing, and muscle cramping in her back. Emotionally, she experienced feelings of anger, irritation, and sadness including instances of unconstrained sobbing. A variety of thoughts, images, and memories surfaced spontaneously.

Occasionally, Hannah would pause the music in order to explain what was happening within her body or to ask for co-regulation. Other times, Heleen would pause the music when she noticed something shift in Hannah's or her own body (through her own neuroception). Heleen would suggest a variety of strategies for Hannah to regulate her state including walking, looking out the window, moving, and supporting herself by pressing her back to a wall. As Hannah felt more comfortable, Heleen would offer touch when appropriate, allowing Hannah the choice to accept or decline.

While some aspects of the music were destabilizing and caused activating sympathetic surges for Hannah, her more common responses were shutdown dorsal reactions. She occasionally slipped into a dissociative state. In these moments, Heleen was able to notice Hannah's state change, stop the music, and support her gently with her voice, touch, and co-regulation to help her to feel that she was not alone.

Summary of Provider's Observations about the Client's Response to SSP

The following is a session-by-session description of what Heleen and Hannah noticed over the five hours of SSP Core.

Session 1, Hour 1 (60 Minutes of Listening)

Hannah was irritated by the music, feeling it was "manipulating" her state. She remarked that if she had been listening to it at home, she would have "tossed it aside 10 times already." Indeed, she needed to pause the music after just three minutes. She was aware of the changes in volume, tempo, and frequencies and felt they activated some old traumatic experiences. Her heart arrhythmias increased. She was dizzy and tended to withdraw into herself as if in a freeze state. She experienced moments when her throat felt closed, and she lost her voice temporarily. Heleen observed Hannah's arousal and tension. She suggested pausing and was able to use her voice and body language to support Hannah in a way that allowed her to resume listening. Hannah was very tired after the session.

Between Sessions

The whole way home, Hannah was both yawning and tearful. She slept deeply that night. In order to be more in contact with her vulnerable parts, Hannah decided to use a breathing ball (Expandaball) in the next sessions.

Session 2, Hour 2 (60 Minutes of Listening)

During this hour, Hannah noticed a woman's laughter in the music, to which she had a sympathetic response wondering, *Is she laughing at me?* and feeling hypervigilant about what might come next. She found that she was silently crying and shaking her head no for much of the session. She also experienced an alternating tightening and relaxing of her throat and jaw and a shortness of breath. Hannah took a few pauses to walk around the room and observe nature through the window and this was calming to her.

Between Sessions

Hannah was somewhat nauseated, had a minor headache, and a desperate need for sweets after the session. That evening she was surprised to notice her shoulders spontaneously drop and relax, a feeling that continued through that night and the next day. Occasionally she noticed some shoulder tension, but the simple thought *This is not necessary* was enough to release the tension.

Session 3, Hour 3 (30 Minutes of Listening)

Hannah experienced the changes in the music as alternating between feelings of hope and harassing activation/insecurity. She felt fortunate to have Heleen witnessing her experience and co-regulating with her. It was during this session and in subsequent ones that Heleen understood that even though she did not know the details of Hannah's trauma history, her "story" wasn't important for their work together. What truly mattered was Heleen being fully present.[*] Hannah, too, could tell that parts of her story were being recalled and were activating to her, but she didn't need to share all the details. Co-regulation was the only thing that was necessary.

Hannah was physically more active during this session. She was swallowing more and could feel her larynx move up and down in her throat. She was also aware of how reactive her jaw was to her emotions. Heleen noticed that Hannah's voice started to change and both her body and her voice became more "grounded."[†]

---

[*] Polyvagal Insight 4: The Power of Social Connection and Co-Regulation

[†] Polyvagal Insight 5: Autonomic State Impacts Social Cues

Between Sessions

After the session, Hannah was very tired and felt cold. She woke up during the night, and her belly hurt. She felt as if there was no hope—only a pervasive sense of being alone and afraid.

Session 4, Hour 3 (30 Minutes of Listening)

Feelings of anger arose during this session as well as some cramping in Hannah's back. Her jaw was reacting, and she cried a little as early memories arose. She allowed Heleen to touch her briefly, providing a physical reminder that she was not alone.

Between Sessions

After the session, Hannah walked her dog and realized that, for the first time in a very long time, she was able to walk for a full hour.

Session 5, Hour 4 (20 Minutes of Listening)

It was helpful for Hannah to stand with her back against a wall during the listening, and she found she could only stand on her left leg. Her throat felt "closed," and she experienced a lot of shaking and shivering. Due to her intense bodily reactions, she couldn't listen much, and they ended the listening early.

Between Sessions

Hannah felt drawn to connect with friends more than she normally would have after the session. She used a punching ball periodically to release her emotions. She also noticed that she felt less alone as she approached the anniversary of her beloved partner's death.

Session 6, Hour 4 (20 Minutes of Listening)

Heleen reported that, while listening, Hannah experienced moments of a deep shutdown response during which she barely made contact. Heleen gradually and carefully moved closer to Hannah until she sensed that she had moved close enough. Using her words and intonation, touch, and presence, Heleen was able to support Hannah back to a balanced ventral vagal state. Hannah expressed a renewed sense of independence and self-sufficiency, feeling capable of managing on her own. She envisioned herself in a pit with a rope beside it, symbolizing her ability to climb out and overcome challenges.

Between Sessions

After the session, Hannah continued to call friends, make plans, and get together with people for lunch. She noticed that her emotions were more fluid—ebbing and flowing like waves. She also began to sense a new physical experience of her own sound resonating in her body, gently trembling in her lips, along the bottom of her mouth, and as a tickling in her chest. She realized she was enjoying exploring these sensations.

Session 7, Hour 4 (20 Minutes of Listening)

Hannah shared that she had been reconnecting with friends and felt her heart more prominently in the front of her body. She was talking more and had a renewed interest in making new plans, something she hadn't felt in years. During the listening, she felt sadness with compassion about how she had held herself back.

Between Sessions

At home, Hannah turned down the radio and television volume as she felt her hearing was better. Her throat also felt more open, and the feeling of her voice resonating within her body continued. She began thinking about organizing more vacations, which she hadn't dared before. And she was becoming more enthusiastic about SSP for both personal and professional reasons.

Session 8, Hour 5 (30 Minutes of Listening)

In conversation during this session, Hannah spoke with growing exuberance and certainty. Heleen noticed that each time they saw each other, Hannah talked and shared much more. She was connected and in a more ventral vagal state. Her voice sounded richer and deeper: it was clear and well-projected, and she could feel it resonating in her body.

---

* Polyvagal Insight 6: Autonomic State, Vocal Intonation, and Middle Ear Muscle Regulation Mutually Influence Each Other

Hannah experienced an epiphany that the higher frequencies of the female voices in the SSP music were particularly activating to her because they resonated with her unmet cries for attachment as a child.

Between Sessions

After the session, Hannah's holiday ended, and her normal work life started again. The switch was not an easy one, and she realized that being "under pressure" drained her energy.* She experienced some diarrhea and a near vasovagal syncope (collapse)—both dorsal vagal withdrawal responses.

Session 9, Hour 5 (30 Minutes of Listening)

Three days after the previous session and despite Hannah's return to the pressures of work, Heleen noticed that Hannah's muscle tension was much lower than the week before. During the listening, Hannah had thoughts such as *I want my life to be about me again* and to her deceased partner, she thought, *You have to let me go.*

Summary of Client's Reflections on Their Response to SSP

Hannah felt SSP was "truly life changing." She was able to shift much more fluidly among her states and was spending more time in a connected ventral vagal state than in a shutdown dorsal one. Many of Hannah's physical complaints like her clenched jaw, groin pain, fatigue, and muscle tension had vanished. She was much more present. Her skin softened and gained color. Her voice returned to its previous lower, richer quality, which she could feel resonating within her body again.†

In the following weeks and months, Hannah felt alive again and that her inner spark had returned. With her therapist, it was possible to work through traumatic experiences that had not been accessible before. Friends and colleagues described her as firmer and steadier, but

---

* Polyvagal Insight 3: Neuroception Detects Cues of Threat and Safety and Alters Autonomic State

† Polyvagal Insight 8: The ANS Is at the Core of Our Physical and Mental Wellness

also softer with a more open and welcoming face.[*] Prior to SSP, Hannah often found herself striving to find a sense of connection and calm, but it wasn't until after SSP that she truly understood what it felt like to be in a ventral vagal state. Once she did, her energy and joy felt completely genuine, radiating outward.

Case Analysis with Dr. Porges

Upon meeting, Heleen and Hannah felt they "spoke the same language" and were immediately at ease with each other, a feeling that grew as they worked together. Hannah appreciated Heleen's quiet but solid, steady, and embodied presence. She trusted and felt safe with her. Without this sense of safety, Hannah would not have had the capacity to be open with Heleen or to new experiences like SSP.

This highlights the importance of neuroception, which refers to the nervous system's continuous scanning and assessing the environment, our relationships, and our own bodies for safety and threat. It is capable of detecting even subtle changes from moment to moment. Heleen consciously respected Hannah's neuroception. She tried to minimize Hannah's reflexive bias to be defensive by building a sense of trust and safety with Hannah at the beginning of each session by asking if she was comfortable and if anything needed to be adjusted. These behavioral sequences provided a platform for their nervous systems to synergistically co-regulate and enabled Hannah to calm and become more accessible.

Heleen also continually assessed how close she could come to Hannah and what kind of eye contact was appropriate and supportive. Hannah frequently looked people in the eyes to gauge the consistency between their words and intentions. She found empty, unengaged eyes triggering, but welcomed the eye contact she had with Heleen. She acknowledged that it was important for her to be seen, but she felt uncomfortable being "looked at." Heleen carefully maintained the just-right approach to allow Hannah's body to reduce its defensiveness

---

[*] Polyvagal Insight 7: The ANS Can Be Retuned to Prioritize Connection and Well-Being

and move toward a connected, ventral vagal state.* This was the foundation for Hannah's openness to SSP.

Voice and Throat Complaints

Two minor issues that resolved for Hannah after SSP were voice constriction and globus pharyngeus. Following SSP, her voice stabilized, and the throat sensation eased significantly, adding to the other benefits she experienced.

Specialists are unable to identify the root cause of physical complaints like these in a substantial percentage of clients. These clients end up being described as having "medically unexplained otorhinolaryngeal symptoms" (MUORLS), which are generally considered to be psychosomatic.

But PVT provides another perspective. Mostly, the pharyngeal and laryngeal muscles involved in speech and sensation in the throat are innervated directly by the vagus nerve, suggesting that low vagal tone may produce vocal impairment and sensory discomfort.† Based on this, Heleen and her research colleague Dr. Keri Heilman provided a neurophysiologically oriented framework to MUORLS by investigating the autonomic features of clients with voice and throat complaints and evaluating the effects of SSP for these features.[1]

They found that clients with voice and throat complaints had significantly poorer autonomic regulation as indicated by higher scores of supradiaphragmatic reactivity on the Body Perception Questionnaire (BPQ) relative to a control group without these complaints. Their research also revealed an improvement in autonomic regulation (lower scores of both supra- and subdiaphragmatic reactivity on the BPQ) following completion of SSP in clients with voice and throat complaints.

And while measures of voice and throat symptomatology were not included in SSP results, it was suggested that the improved autonomic regulation following SSP would enable clients with voice and throat

---

* Polyvagal Insight 3: Neuroception Detects Cues of Threat and Safety and Alters Autonomic State

† Polyvagal Insight 8: The ANS Is at the Core of Our Physical and Mental Wellness

complaints to be more receptive to treatments or interventions. This provides optimism and new directions to support those with MUORLS.

With improved autonomic regulation, the vagus nerve can function optimally. Hannah's journey shows that voice and throat complaints can abate without any targeted speech therapy or ear, nose, and throat interventions. For her, the improvement in autonomic regulation alone was enough to eliminate her symptoms.

Physical and Emotional Responses

Early in the listening, Hannah experienced physical symptoms like stomach tightness, heart arrhythmia, and muscle tension, along with emotional responses like anger, irritation, and sadness. These initial reactions suggest that SSP was actively engaging Hannah's ANS. When these sensations and emotions arose, Heleen was able to sensitively attune, pace, and process them with Hannah. Paradoxically, dramatic early responses like Hannah's are often a good indicator of the potential for an overall positive outcome with SSP.

Hannah also experienced intense bodily reactions like shaking and shivering during SSP listening. She noticed this particularly during Hour 4 of SSP when the frequency range of the filtered music is widened and there are times when the frequencies of the human voice disappear. Hannah was likely experiencing temporary shifts out of a ventral vagal state and into a sympathetic one. The shaking and shivering are adaptive sympathetic responses. She also experienced nausea between sessions, which may have resulted from a dorsal vagal reaction.

Responses to the Frequencies of SSP

Initially, Hannah felt that she was being manipulated by the music. She expressed her discomfort as she became aware of it and felt comfortable enough to say when she needed to pause the music due to a bodily sensation. This occurred during Hannah's first listening session after just three minutes. Heleen supported her by addressing the issue directly and handling it straightforwardly.

Gradually, Hannah came to experience the music not as manipulation but as an invitation to experience a felt sense of safety in her body.

As she listened, her nervous system shifted between defensive and connected physiological states. This frequent transitioning among states improved her capacity to move fluidly along her autonomic continuum. She also began to recognize the sensations, thoughts, emotions, and behaviors associated with her connected ventral state, which gave her the opportunity to intentionally develop skills to help her move into that state more readily. Hannah's rekindled joy in spending time with friends, along with her restored inner spark and sense of vitality, reflect the improved balance and flexibility of her ANS.

Implications for Daily Life

A notable portion of all healthcare encounters, ranging from 20 to 45 percent,[2] are characterized by persistent bodily and functional symptoms that lack an obvious cause or recognized mechanism despite thorough medical investigation. These include MUORLS, chronic pain and fatigue, and irritable bowel syndrome, among others. Recognizing how the ANS influences these unexplained symptoms is key to initiating healing and recovery.

Traditional medical approaches typically focus on treating the specific organ where symptoms manifest. In contrast, polyvagal theory takes a more integrated approach. It emphasizes the role of the entire system rather than just the affected organ. A dysregulated nervous system can cause multiple organs and systems to function suboptimally. If an organ shows no clear signs of injury or disease but still causes symptoms, the root cause may be a dysregulated nervous system. The good news is that techniques like SSP can retune the ANS and enhance vagal regulation to support holistic healing and an overall better quality of life.

Chapter 7

From Chronic Pain and Hearing Loss to Healing, Hope, and Joy

Case Overview

> **SSP PROVIDER:** Autum Romano, LMT, CNMT, CST, Reiki master. Website: autumromano.com
>
> **CLINICAL DISCIPLINE AND FOCUS:** Educator, bodyworker, and author passionate about nervous system regulation as a foundation for transformative whole health
>
> **OTHER THERAPEUTIC MODALITIES AND EXPERTISE:** Neuromuscular therapy, massage therapy, myofascial release, craniosacral therapy, cupping therapy, Reiki, and PVT
>
> **CLIENT:** Naomi, a woman in her early 30s, sought out Autum's massage therapy after searching for relief from her chronic pain and exploring various other treatments. Her experience was so impactful that she quit her job as an office manager, enrolled in massage school, and is now a massage therapist and SSP provider. Website: naomimassagetherapy.com
>
> **FEATURES/SYMPTOMS:** History of early and long-term abuse; extreme hypersensitivities; cyclical ear infections and episodes of hearing loss; long-term experience of periodic vomiting and fainting; and chronic pain

AUTONOMIC TENDENCY: Naomi often experienced a freeze state in which she exhibited low facial affect but high tension in her trunk and neck. Sometimes she oscillated between sympathetic and dorsal vagal states in a cyclic defense loop.

ASSESSMENTS: Beyond Autum's standard intake process and measures, no formal assessments were utilized.

Client Description

From an early age through young adulthood, Naomi and her sister Anna were sexually and emotionally abused by people who should have been trustworthy. Despite being only four years older, Anna protected and supported Naomi. Their sisterly bond provided them with a sense of secure attachment, although neither experienced enough autonomy or agency to change their situation.

Starting at age 10, Naomi experienced numerous ear disorders including difficulty equalizing the air pressure in her ears, ear pain, periods of deafness in her left ear, and tinnitus. In her teen years, Naomi experienced frequent fainting and vomiting, which drew unwanted attention from her peers. The fainting ended when Naomi was in her early 20s when she gained independence from her family and the vomiting stopped after she moved into a new home with her partner Joshua several years later.* By the time she met Autum in her early 30s, Naomi's most prominent symptom was chronic pain.

Before meeting Autum, Naomi had scoured the traditional medicine world seeing many different doctors without finding relief from her persistent neck, back, head, and ear pain. When she was medically diagnosed with fibromyalgia at age 21, she felt it was "the end of a sentence instead of the beginning of a question." She firmly believed her multiple symptoms had a common source and that, somehow, she would find an answer—or at least a better question to ask. Despite her ongoing symptoms and challenges, she maintained a sense of hope and curiosity as she navigated her own path toward wellness.

---

* Polyvagal Insight 8: The ANS Is at the Core of Our Physical and Mental Wellness

Nearly a decade later, Naomi was still searching for relief from her pain and was open to new approaches. She met Autum at a neurofeedback clinic where Naomi worked and learned about Autum's massage and neuromuscular therapy work.

SSP Delivery Method

Autum and Naomi met monthly for the first year of working together and later shifted to every other week. Initially, Autum only used Reiki, myofascial release, and neuromuscular therapy with Naomi while they were building a strong foundation together. Naomi's soft tissue felt rigid and defensive in the initial sessions. Naomi responded well to deep tissue trigger point work and preferred intensive manual therapy. Autum was reluctant to use that much pressure but, at the time, it was the only input Naomi's body could receive and process. At this point, Naomi was only aware of some aspects of her trauma history; she did not yet understand its full extent or that her pain could be a result of it.

Autum began teaching Naomi about PVT and physiological states. She used "green," "red," and "blue" to describe the three primary states (ventral vagal, sympathetic, and dorsal vagal). Naomi was keenly interested and soon they were sharing insights into the theory, their own autonomic tendencies, and their observations.

After several months, Autum suggested SSP to Naomi, and she agreed to integrate it into their sessions. Autum used 30–60 minutes of SSP Core at the beginning of every session to help prepare Naomi's body for massage therapy. In response, Naomi's back pain began to decrease and her neck, head, and ear pain became the focus of Autum's targeted manual therapy.

After Naomi finished the five hours of SSP Core, she listened to Hours 3, 4, and 5 again during their sessions to prolong the effects of SSP. She began each session lying face down on the table so Autum could work on her back and listened with headphones. Autum used Reiki, neuromuscular therapy, myofascial release, craniosacral therapy, and therapeutic massage as appropriate for Naomi's autonomic state at the moment. The headphones were removed when Naomi rolled to her back.

Naomi's SSP listening experience validated the importance of the adage "safe before sound." Having a trusting connection with Autum and with her co-regulation, Naomi easily absorbed the input of SSP. After Naomi completed eight hours of SSP listening during their sessions, Autum recommended that Naomi could do some listening on her own. However, Naomi found it difficult and more activating than when they were together. Autum suggested that she hold hands with Joshua while listening. That safe physical connection enabled Naomi's nervous system to receive the music. Over time, Naomi consistently found that holding Joshua's hand or sitting with one of her dogs enhanced her response to SSP.*

After completing SSP Core a second time, Naomi began to use Hour 4 or 5 of SSP Core as a way of addressing her periodic bouts of severe ear and neck pain. She then moved to listening to SSP Balance and found that it relieved her pain and that she could listen to it for longer time spans while on her own than she could to SSP Core.

As Naomi accessed her green state more easily, she became better able to accept manual therapy, and her receptivity to touch increased. Her autonomic state was the key factor that maximized the benefits she gained from massage therapy,† and when Autum could read and track the state of Naomi's body and match her technique to Naomi's state, the session was more successful, and Naomi's specific pains were relieved.

Summary of Provider's Observations about the Client's Response to SSP

The most fundamental change that resulted from Autum's work with Naomi was that Naomi's body and nervous system learned to feel safe.

Gradually, Naomi became able to string together moments of "green," and this allowed her body to shift out of her previous experience of pain as a permanent way of living. Through this process and with the help

---

* Polyvagal Insight 4: The Power of Social Connection and Co-Regulation

† Polyvagal Insight 3: Neuroception Detects Cues of Threat and Safety and Alters Autonomic State

of SSP, Naomi began to discover how to inhabit her body. She came to realize that for most of her life, she felt like a "brain driving a human-shaped vehicle around," but now she felt like her brain and body were connected.

Autum believed that bodywork could repair attachment wounds, especially when clients were able to access the blended state of safety with immobilization (green and blue states) for the duration of their sessions. As if to prove this, Naomi and Joshua's relationship grew in tandem with Naomi's nervous system healing. Naomi's in-office work with Autum created enough safety in Naomi's body that her nervous system could experience deeper safety with Joshua. Naomi credited Autum, Joshua, and her sister Anna with demonstrating to her that relationships could be safe and nurturing.

As Naomi responded to Autum's touch with greater softening and attunement, her chronic pain lessened, leading to reduced discomfort and improved fluidity in her movement. With each session, Autum was able to use increasingly less force and a lighter touch, still relying on neuromuscular therapy to unlock the cervical spine and occiput but also using myofascial release and craniosacral therapy.

As a result of the combination of SSP and manual therapy, Autum could feel Naomi's occiput and cervical vertebrae spontaneously mobilize and shift in every session. Memories surfaced during sessions, and it was clear that integration was happening. Naomi's facial expressivity would shift from flat to animated, and her vocal quality became richer and warmer after a session.[*] Her neck also transitioned from being guarded and stiff to trusting and supple, making it easier to work with her cervical spine. Naomi's ear pain would be relieved after a session, and her breathing would settle into a slower, deeper pace. She became progressively more aware of the effects of her autonomic shifts. Where previously, defensive states would feel "wrong" and sometimes lead to a downward spiral, she began to see her state changes as normal.

---

[*] Polyvagal Insight 5: Autonomic State Impacts Social Cues

She accepted that she could get stuck in defensive states but also now knew ways to shift out of them.

Naomi was an astute observer of herself and was able to give explicit feedback to Autum, which allowed the progress to continue. This was unusual for someone with a trauma background and chronic pain, but Naomi had the capacity to trust and stay attuned to her physical sensations. Naomi's awe at her personal response to her work with Autum inspired her to invest in herself and enroll in massage school.

The supportive relationship between Autum and Naomi was an essential component of Naomi's therapy. By the second year, the two had developed a deep bond and a shared curiosity and wonder about Naomi's various responses and how they related to her body and nervous system. The healing process was one of exploration and joint decision-making—especially as Naomi grew in self-awareness and intuitiveness and made progress in massage school and in her own study of PVT.

Naomi's ability to access and remain in her green state increased continuously. As Autum put it, "When we were working together in green, there was a fluid and deep resonance between us that pulsed with the rhythm of connection."*

Summary of Client's Reflections on Their Response to SSP

To Naomi, SSP, bodywork, and co-regulation were her medicine. They alleviated her pain and helped her unwind unhelpful nervous system patterns. Without these interventions, Naomi was sure she would have had to visit the emergency room multiple times due to her pain. After two years of working with Autum, so much had transformed in her body and nervous system that her fibromyalgia seemed like a distant memory.

Before SSP, Naomi's pain level usually moved between 5 and 8 on a scale of 1 to 10. Some days, it would move up to a 9 or 10 and a few times her pain dipped below 5. On these "below 5" days, she felt hope for the chance of a pain-free life. After SSP, her daily pain level was

* Polyvagal Insight 4: The Power of Social Connection and Co-Regulation

between 0 and 3. Infrequently, it would go up to a 5 and very rarely, it would go above that.

Once, when they were working with acute pain, Naomi found it very difficult to bear. Autum suggested that she "lean into rather than pulling away from the pain." This phrasing resonated with Naomi, providing a helpful insight that initiated a significant change in her approach to life. Instead of running from her red activated state where she experienced her most pain and aggravation, she started accepting it and then could shift her state. Where her red state had once been frightening and associated with "bad things happening," she could endure it more easily. And her blue state no longer seemed like a hopeless life sentence.

Naomi's enhanced autonomic flexibility significantly altered her receptivity to touch. Despite her lifelong extreme hypersensitivity to sensory experiences, being held in Autum's supportive green state allowed Naomi to access her own green state, and she became more receptive to physical touch. Her body became more pliable, enabling the massage work to be more effective with less pressure. Naomi recognized that major mobilizations of her joints and soft tissue were achievable when she was in her green state. Conversely, when her body was in a defensive state, it was more guarded and challenging to work with.[*]

Her capacity to handle stressors with ease increased. In her second year of treatment, in the span of one week, her dog died, a close relative was hospitalized, she was in a car accident, and Joshua's motorcycle was stolen. She was able to remain resilient and avoid dropping into her blue state, thus preventing feelings of overwhelm and despondency. Her story was not "Bad things are happening to me" but instead, "A lot is happening at the same time, and it is a lot to manage."

Naomi's associations with the music of SSP were so positive that she came to love the songs on the SSP Core playlist despite them being outside her natural musical preferences. Her system *wanted* to listen to this music and, in difficult situations, she found herself conjuring the music in her head. Although surprising to her at first, she came to rely on her

---

[*] Polyvagal Insight 2: Autonomic States Bias Our Feelings, Thoughts, and Behaviors

musical memory to help regulate her behaviors, thoughts, and emotions in the moment.

Naomi was finally able to identify the common factor among her symptoms as the state of her nervous system.* In her words, "Things happened to me and they seemed unexplainable until now." After two years of working with Autum, Naomi had made significant changes in her life. She left her steady job, attended massage school, started her own massage therapy business, and became an SSP provider herself. She felt great satisfaction as her life filled with joy and meaning.

Naomi recognized Anna, her sister, and Joshua as steady co-regulators crucial to her personal transformation. Through PVT, SSP, and her work with Autum, Naomi was able to cultivate a safer, happier self, emerging triumphantly from the trauma and chronic pain she had endured.

Case Analysis with Dr. Porges

Naomi's comment that her diagnosis of fibromyalgia felt like "the end of a sentence instead of the beginning of a question" is poignant. Diagnoses are just labels and without an understanding of mechanism, they will lead to unreliable treatment models and poor outcomes. We now know far more about the body and nervous system and can use this to inform and change the way we approach the treatment of many conditions. There can be a tendency for medical providers to rush in and try to directly fix problems, rather than recognizing the importance of allowing—and actively supporting—the body's natural healing processes. Healing begins when the body receives signals that it no longer needs to remain in a defensive state. Effective therapies, such as those Naomi received, facilitated this process. The body is intelligent and works in our favor when given the right support.

This confirms what we've known since Walter Hess's 1949 Nobel prize lecture[1] that all systems in the body are intertwined to support the self-regulation of bodily organs or "homeostasis," a term coined by

---

* Polyvagal Insight 8: The ANS Is at the Core of Our Physical and Mental Wellness

Walter Cannon[2] as a modern update of Claude Bernard's concept of "internal milieu."[3]

A Constellation of Symptoms

Thinking holistically, it's possible to view Naomi's symptoms of chronic pain, ear disorders, fainting, and gut issues as resulting from disruptions of the ANS. The literature links nonspecific chronic disorders like fibromyalgia and irritable bowel syndrome with the ANS being locked in defense.[4] Initially, sympathetic responses support strategies like hypersensitivities and pain. When these sympathetic responses failed to move Naomi into safety, dorsal vagal pathways triggered fainting. Poor vagal regulation not only heightens sympathetic reactivity but also facilitates fainting as a dorsal vagal reflexive defense. This undermines access to ventral vagal influences that would support the homeostatic processes leading to optimal health and trusting co-regulatory relationships.

In response to her early life experiences, Naomi's nervous system adapted by prioritizing protective defensive pathways over co-regulatory connecting pathways to cope with her constant experience of extreme threat. While it helped her to survive, it led to a disruption in homeostatic processes. Living in a state of chronic defensiveness increases our risk of eventually developing symptoms of chronic illnesses.

Chronic Pain

Acute pain serves as a clear signal of threat, prompting the body to take immediate action. In contrast, chronic pain involves sympathetic hypervigilance, where the brain and body remain trapped in a persistent state of threat. This ongoing state primes the body for self-protection, with pain signaling the need for attention and safeguarding. Naomi insightfully wondered if pain might be her body's way of reaching out for safety and connection.

Bodywork with Autum began the process of gently unwinding Naomi's nervous system patterns and addressing her pain. Initially, Naomi's body required deep and intensive manual therapy with a lot of pressure. She was experiencing numbness and a limited awareness of bodily feelings, a natural response to being locked in a chronic state of defense. Trauma often leads to numbness and a blurred boundaries. Naomi was seeking those boundaries. Autum's firm pressure helped Naomi define and reconnect with the edges of her body. Similarly, the pressure of a weighted blanket provides cues of where the body ends.

Courageously, Naomi sought to be assured that people weren't dangerous and wouldn't hurt her. Although she knew she was no longer in immediate danger, her pain remained a subconscious reminder of her previous experience of extreme threat and vulnerability. A natural strategy would have been not to venture out again. But at our core, we all need human connection; that biological imperative never goes away. Autum worked respectfully and collaboratively and was able to earn Naomi's trust—not only with her words but with her intentions, skill, curiosity, and steadfastness. Over time, Naomi's body and nervous system felt safe enough to turn off its defenses. The pain released its grip, and her body began to express its own rhythms of homeostasis.

Ear Disorders

Frequent ear infections are often associated with auditory hypersensitivity and deficits in auditory and language processing. These infections may result from poor functioning of the eustachian tubes, which link the middle ear to the throat, helping regulate the air pressure in the ears. The middle ear muscles, especially the tensor tympani, which is innervated by the trigeminal nerve (CN V), one of the cranial nerves involved in the SES, helps open and close the eustachian tubes. If the eustachian tubes remain closed due to a dysregulated nervous system and low vagal tone, mucus can build up in the middle ear, which can cause ear infection symptoms.

Equalization problems in the ears can also indicate issues with the middle ear muscles, and symptoms may include pain, balance problems or dizziness, a feeling of fullness in the ear or ears, and/or distorted hearing.

Tinnitus is the perception of noise or ringing in the ears without an external sound source. It is a relatively common but distressing condition, and research is ongoing. One hypothesis is that it may result from a reduction in the functions of the ventral vagal complex. It could also be linked to the presence of an acoustic neuroma or inflammation of the auditory nerve. Additionally, tinnitus may worsen due to stress or low vagal tone. As in Naomi's case, where her symptoms of tinnitus were significantly reduced, SSP has been demonstrated to reduce the response to tinnitus in some individuals through improved vagal tone.

When the SES is retracted and the body shifts into a defensive state, neural tone to the middle ear muscles is reduced. This can increase susceptibility to ear infections, equalization problems, and potentially, tinnitus.*

There is a close neurophysiological relationship between the neural regulation of the vagus and the neural regulation of the muscles of the face and head, including the middle ear muscles. Thus, poor vagal regulation of the autonomic nervous system is often comorbid with a depressed social engagement system including structures related via the ventral complex (e.g., a flat facial affect, a lack of prosody in the voice, and auditory hypersensitivities).

A Double Legacy

Naomi's older sister Anna gave her the early experience of a safe refuge. But that existed within a broader landscape of inescapable threat for both of them. Naomi emerged as an adult with a double legacy. One part of her had strength and a positive, hopeful outlook derived from her nervous system's experience of foundational safety with Anna. This gave her the inner resources to steer clear of powerful pain medications and instead to find an understanding partner and supportive healer. Meanwhile, another part of Naomi's nervous system was still trapped in a state of threat expressed as physical pain and rigidity. Autum's support and Joshua's connection enabled that part of Naomi to gradually soften, to recognize that the old threat was gone, and to feel safe.

---

* Polyvagal Insight 6: Autonomic State, Vocal Intonation, and Middle Ear Muscle Regulation Mutually Influence Each Other

Implications for Daily Life

Safe and co-regulatory relationships are essential for well-being, contributing to a fulfilling and balanced life and even longevity. However, for individuals with a trauma history, forming such connections can be challenging because the damage has been within close relationships, which should have been safe and nurturing. These individuals require abundant and explicit signals of safety to build trust and activate their SES. Key elements in fostering a sense of safety for meaningful connection include respect, authenticity, patience, and commitment.

Chapter 8

Tormented Teen Gets Her Life Back

Case Overview

SSP PROVIDER: Doreen Hunt, MA, OTR/L, co-owner of Children's Therapy of Woodinville. Website: childrenstherapyofwoodinville.com/doreen-hunt-ma-otr-l/

CLINICAL DISCIPLINE AND FOCUS: Occupational therapy with a focus on pediatrics and specializing in sensory processing, auditory processing disorders, nervous system health, and trauma-informed care

OTHER THERAPEUTIC MODALITIES AND EXPERTISE: Sensory integration therapy and the Total Focus System sound and movement therapy

CLIENT: Ruth (a pseudonym) is a 16-year-old with a history of academic stress, anxiety, and depression. She experienced panic attacks, self-harm, hallucinations, and two suicide attempts during the prior year and a half.

FEATURES/SYMPTOMS: Hypersensitivities (auditory, tactile, and vestibular), ADHD, dyscalculia, anxiety, depression, panic attacks, body and facial tension, frequent elevated heart rate, auditory and visual hallucinations, self-harm, and suicidality

AUTONOMIC TENDENCY: The cyclic defense loop, an oscillation between sympathetic and dorsal vagal states

ASSESSMENTS: SCAN-3:A Test for Auditory Processing Disorders in Adolescents and Adults (three subtests), and the Autonomic Resilience Screener (ANS Screener)

Client Description

On the outside, Ruth appeared to be a warm and composed teenager. She enjoyed spending time with friends, working out at the gym, playing lacrosse for her high school team, painting, and engaging in creative arts and music. However, beneath the surface, she was caught in a cyclic defense loop of anxiety and depression.

In school, she got good grades, but it took a lot of hard work and perseverance as well as second chances from her teachers. She felt tremendous pressure from all sides to excel, but there were times when even her hardest efforts weren't enough. As far back as the 1st and 2nd grades, between the ages of 6 and 7, she had struggled with math and reading and saw a tutor during the school year and every summer. When she was in 6th grade, at age 11, her parents separated and eventually divorced.

By 8th grade, at age 13, Ruth's mother found her crying in her closet and realized it was time to seek outside help. A neuropsychological examination revealed that Ruth had difficulties with attentional control, executive functions, and coping with stress. Toward the end of 8th grade, Ruth started seeing a psychotherapist, and an education support plan was established at school.

COVID significantly disrupted Ruth's life. While academics became less demanding with everything moving online during 9th grade—resulting in fewer tests and reduced pressure—the social impact was more challenging. Being isolated from her friends and missing the entire season of lacrosse, a sport she loved and a key way she connected with others, left her feeling disconnected and deprived of the camaraderie that was so important to her.

In the summer before 10th grade, at age 15, Ruth was self-harming, a behavior she later revealed began in 7th grade, when she was 12. She had stopped seeing the therapist from 8th grade and requested to find someone new. Things took a turn for the worse when school resumed in person for the first time in a year and a half. Ruth started hearing a male voice in her head telling her to hurt herself, and sometimes, she even "saw" him. A few months into the fall, she attempted suicide.

Her therapist provided solid support and prescribed antidepressants. However, shortly afterward, her panic attacks worsened to the point where she had to leave school temporarily and enroll in an intensive six-week partial hospitalization program. While she learned some helpful dialectical behavioral therapy (DBT) skills there, Ruth continued to struggle with depression, severe anxiety, and frequent panic attacks.

The following summer, just before 11th grade at age 16, Ruth attempted suicide again. In November, she self-harmed severely enough to require emergency room treatment. Her parents were deeply concerned, worrying not *if* but *when* she would harm herself again. Desperate for help, her mother researched out-of-state residential facilities. Although Ruth hated the idea of being away from her family and friends for months, she would do anything to escape the pain she was experiencing.

During that stressful and terrifying time, Ruth's mom received a recommendation from a friend whose daughter had achieved remarkable results from sound therapy years earlier. The friend highly recommended working with Doreen Hunt. Although neither Ruth nor her mom fully understood what SSP was, they were willing to try anything that might help.

SSP Delivery Method

Recognizing the severity of Ruth's condition and history, as well as her strong motivation to heal, Doreen believed that SSP could be beneficial. She was also reassured by the fact that Ruth had a very supportive family and the guidance of a skilled psychotherapist.

On the ANS Screener Doreen used as part of her intake process, Ruth reported numerous hypersensitivities, such as irritation from certain fabrics, motion sickness, and constant distraction by sound making it difficult to follow verbal instructions in noisy environments. Physically, Ruth reported regular tension in her body and face, dizziness, fidgetiness, a rapid heart rate, and fatigue. Emotionally, Ruth felt angry, irritable, lonely, overwhelmed, and anxious, and she was reluctant to engage in social activities about 50 percent of the time. She also struggled with frequent inattention, racing thoughts, memory issues, difficulty understanding text, challenges with verbal communication, and trouble starting or completing tasks.

During their first meeting, Doreen explained the nervous system and PVT to Ruth and her mom. This helped them understand that Ruth was likely trapped in an autonomic cycle between sympathetic activation (characterized by stress, anxiety, and body tension) and dorsal disconnection (marked by depression, frequent fatigue, and hopelessness). Eager to feel the connected ventral vagal state Doreen described, Ruth listened to the first 30 minutes of SSP Core alongside Doreen in the clinic. She enjoyed the session and was pleased to find that the SSP music included songs she knew.

Because Ruth felt comfortable at home with her mother and had access to Doreen and her psychotherapist, Doreen recommended that Ruth listen to 30 minutes of SSP Core each day with her mom. After the second day, Ruth reported feeling "super tired" and needing to take a nap both days. Although she felt "more connected to herself," she also experienced a degree of being overwhelmed. Doreen suggested reducing the listening time to 15 minutes a day, which proved to be a more manageable pace for Ruth. While she listened, Ruth engaged in calming activities like painting with watercolors, playing solitaire, or organizing her room. She found the listening experience to be soothing and even expressed a desire for the music to continue, saying she "wished it didn't stop." Ruth completed the five hours of SSP Core over three weeks. After a short break, she repeated Hours 3, 4, and 5 by listening for 30 minutes each day to reinforce the benefits she had experienced.

Now, Ruth listens to SSP Balance about three to four times a week. She finds that when she feels overwhelmed, just 15 minutes of listening helps to calm and settle her.

Summary of Provider's Observations about the Client's Response to SSP

When her mom suggested trying yet another approach, Ruth was skeptical because she thought SSP sounded "weird." However, she was still willing to try it because she was "desperate to find a way to cope with her depression and anxiety." She also hoped it would help her "reduce her bad thoughts and improve her motivation."

Doreen's short-term goals were for Ruth to feel safer, increase her happiness, and access her calm and connected ventral vagal state more easily. Long-term, the aims were improved attention, better self-regulation, and reduced disruptions from hypersensitivities. Not only were these goals met and exceeded, but Ruth also reported significant improvements: her body tension and her repetitive thoughts diminished from "almost always" to "almost never," and her sense of feeling distant from others improved from "frequently" to "rarely."

While not everyone experiences it this way, Ruth felt the effects of SSP almost immediately. For the first time in many months, she felt "a weight come off her shoulders." Doreen noted that, as a clinician, you don't always grasp the full extent of your client's story, especially early in the therapeutic relationship, until safety is established. Initially, Ruth did not disclose that she suffered from almost daily auditory and/or visual hallucinations urging her to self-harm and commit suicide. It was profound when she later revealed that after listening to just the first 30 minutes of SSP Core, she completely stopped seeing or hearing the man's voice in her head. When Doreen suggested slowing down the listening, Ruth feared the voice would return, but it didn't, and it hasn't. Even after six months, Ruth had still not heard the man's voice or seen him since before those initial 30 minutes of SSP.

As Ruth continued with SSP, she began to regain her energy and noticed a significant and rapid decrease in her anxiety. She described that "everything became more comfortable to live with." When she transitioned to listening to SSP Balance, she felt "more put together" with her thoughts and feelings becoming more balanced. To Doreen, Ruth appeared more stable, with reduced anxiety, greater social engagement, and improved executive functioning. She also seemed happier, with a quicker smile and more eye contact.[*]

Exuberant about her results and ever thoughtful about those around her, Ruth is now wondering how some of her friends might access SSP. She believes it could help so many people.

Assessments

The SCAN-3 test assesses an individual's auditory processing abilities, including their ability to focus on specific sounds amid background noise, process rapid speech, selectively listen in challenging situations, and retain and recall auditory information. These auditory processing skills significantly impact attention and executive functioning skills. And sensitivity to sound and loud environments can be a symptom of people experiencing stress.

Pre-SSP, Ruth's auditory processing skills appeared within low normal levels on three subtests. But Ruth's left ear scores were below the typical range on three subtests. After SSP, this improved to be within normal limits on two of the three subtests.

Post-SSP, her ability to focus on and extract relevant auditory information while filtering out irrelevant background sounds (Auditory Figure Ground subtest) and her ability to process a fast rate of speech (Time Compressed Sentences subtest) improved considerably. Additionally, an audiologist completed a full central auditory processing assessment one month post-SSP, and Ruth's results were all within normal limits.

Summary of Client's and Parents' Reflections on Client's Response to SSP

The primary hope for SSP was that Ruth would rediscover a sense of hope, find relief from the weight of self-harm and suicidal thoughts, and ultimately embrace life with joy and vitality. Remarkably, from the very first SSP Core listening session, Ruth stopped hearing the voice that

---

[*] Polyvagal Insight 8: The ANS Is at the Core of Our Physical and Mental Wellness

urged her to hurt herself, and it hasn't returned. There were no greater goals than ensuring Ruth's safety and happiness.

Early on, her father noticed changes in her demeanor, facial expression, and voice. Her face was more relaxed, her eyes seemed brighter, and she had better eye contact. The quality of her voice changed, and it became more energetic. He also felt that even how she moved and held her body seemed different—her pace quickened, and she seemed to do things more purposefully.[*]

Ruth's mother noticed a rapid transformation in Ruth; she became noticeably more relaxed and happy and exuded genuine calmness. She also observed that Ruth's anxiety seemed to decrease. Ruth appeared to be "happy to be living rather than just making it through the day exhausted, moving from one thing to the next." Her mother was "amazed by what SSP did and continues to do for her." She called SSP a "miracle" because they were ready to send Ruth out of state for a treatment program. Now, she describes Ruth as a joyful teenager leading a busy life, enjoying everything.

Ruth feels that SSP definitely changed her life for the better. It gave her the necessary foundation to embrace healthy coping mechanisms and safeguard her mental health. She is now able to handle the stress of school much better and she continues to feel and do so much better. Ruth and her parents recognized that she was at a dangerous crossroads where things could have gone very badly, but luckily a path toward SSP was found.

Case Analysis with Dr. Porges

This case highlights the significant impact SSP can have on altering a young person's life trajectory and its positive effects on their family. Ruth's ANS Screener responses suggested underlying ANS dysregulation and hypersensitivities to auditory, tactile, and vestibular stimuli, along with challenges such as ADHD and dyscalculia that had previously gone unrecognized, affecting her cognitive skills. The relationship between

---

[*] Polyvagal Insight 5: Autonomic State Impacts Social Cues

ANS dysregulation and these conditions created a "chicken and egg" scenario, making it hard to determine whether dysregulation led to these conditions, or if the conditions exacerbated the dysregulation. A dysregulated nervous system can cause considerable distress, including anxiety, depression, panic attacks, self-harm, and even suicidality.

When considering SSP for sensitive cases like Ruth's, it is important to establish a strong safety net and proceed with careful consideration. Creating the "safe before sound" involves establishing the most supportive conditions to maximize the effectiveness of SSP. This requires attention to the client's state, setting, and support in their life.

First, working with a highly experienced SSP provider is essential. The provider should collaborate with a therapist who has the relevant scope of practice to monitor progress and offer support if the SSP provider does not have this specialty themselves. Second, the client must have a safe and stable living situation with a trusted person who is aware of their circumstances and will regularly check in on them. Third, the provider must thoroughly understand the client's experience, background, and nervous system to anticipate and address needs both initially and as the process unfolds.

Doreen's intake process with Ruth exemplifies this approach, and a specific SSP Intake Form is available to support it. Doreen was careful to understand all aspects of Ruth's situation. Gaining a comprehensive understanding of the client's situation, including elements that may not be immediately obvious, is critical for providing effective support and ensuring SSP is both safe and beneficial. This case also underscores the value for some clients of ongoing SSP use for maintaining progress and preventing regression into previous patterns of distress.

Evaluative Environments and Academic Stress

Evaluations are fundamental to the educational system, but while some students excel under pressure, high-stakes evaluative situations can be threatening for many, triggering survival states that compromise executive functioning and hinder performance. Executive functions are higher cognitive processes that enable goal setting, planning, initiating actions, impulse control, and self-regulation. They also include working memory, attention, and problem-solving skills. When a person perceives a threat, their access to these cognitive functions can be compromised, creating a feedback loop where stress from evaluation worsens performance issues. This increased pressure can lead to further difficulties with schoolwork.

The fear of being assessed or judged can push the ANS into a defensive state, which can manifest as either hyperactivation or overwhelm.* In Ruth's case, she became stuck in a cyclic defense loop, which sometimes resulted in anxiety and panic about school (sympathetic activation) and other times led to a sense of being overwhelmed and unsure of where to begin (dorsal vagal shutdown).† Each state is metabolically costly, and so the individual toggles between the two when either one becomes too taxing. The relentless oscillation between these states led to symptoms that necessitated the use of both antidepressants and antianxiety medication.

Ruth's intense anxiety is not an isolated experience but rather reflects a broader trend seen among many of her peers. The effects of social media, reduced face-to-face interactions, and the impact of social isolation due to the COVID pandemic and other factors may be contributing to rising mental health challenges among teenagers. According to survey data from the US Centers for Disease Control and Prevention, rates of high schoolers feeling persistently sad or hopeless increased from one in four in 2011 to nearly one in two by 2021. During the same decade, emergency room visits for anxiety, mood disorders, eating disorders, and self-harm increased, and suicide rates soared.[1]

Auditory Processing and Hypersensitivities

Ruth's SCAN-3 testing and personal experiences revealed challenges in focusing on speech amid background noise. This could be caused by a chronic defensive state; in threatening situations, neural networks associated with listening prioritize lower and higher frequency ranges, which

---

* Polyvagal Insight 3: Neuroception Detects Cues of Threat and Safety and Alters Autonomic State

† Polyvagal Insight 2: Autonomic States Bias Our Feelings, Thoughts, and Behaviors

are evolutionarily associated with danger and alertness.* The emphasis on these frequency bands instead of on the frequency range of the human voice can obscure voices, making them harder to discern.

An impaired ability to understand speech significantly affects one's quality of life, leading to communication challenges, misunderstandings, cognitive strain, and emotional impacts such as social withdrawal, frustration, and diminished confidence. Difficulty understanding speech is also experienced in age-related hearing loss where, over time, we can develop difficulty in deciphering speech amid background noise.

SSP addresses auditory processing deficiencies by delivering cues of safety. When the brainstem receives these signals of safety, it relays instructions, via branches of the trigeminal, facial, and vagus nerves, to the muscles of the middle ear, which enhance the extraction of the middle frequencies of voice.[2] Our nervous system loves the intonation of voice, and we are soothed by its melody. Research has shown that vocal prosody is associated with decreases in infant distress and improvement in infant autonomic regulation.[3]

When our physiology is driven by defensiveness, our perception of threat signals is amplified. This heightened state can increase sensitivities to sound, tactile sensations, and vestibular signals like motion sickness. Biological cues like hunger can quickly escalate into "hanger" when emotions are intensified by physiological needs.†

These sensory and biological triggers are inherent to all of us, often leading to reactivity without full awareness. Additionally, our physiological responses can unintentionally trigger similar reactions in others.

SSP offers a method to mitigate these threat reactions by delivering signals of safety. These inputs guided Ruth's physiological state to repeatedly shift from heightened activation or shutdown toward a connected state during SSP sessions. This neural exercise helped to repattern her nervous system to have greater access to her ventral vagal complex.

---

* Polyvagal Insight 6: Autonomic State, Vocal Intonation, and Middle Ear Muscle Regulation Mutually Influence Each Other

† Polyvagal Insight 1: Autonomic State Functions as an Intervening Variable

As a result of this repatterning, Ruth experienced various improvements. She started craving and enjoying social connections with friends again. She noticed reduced bodily tension, fewer intrusive thoughts, and a significantly diminished anxiety around test taking. Notably, her SCAN-3 scores improved, indicating a restoration in her ability to accurately process incoming sounds.*

Hallucinations, Self-Harm, and Suicide Attempts

When we become trapped in a cyclic defense loop, we're numb, and we can't listen to what our body is telling us. We may become defensive toward others and experience hypersensitivities. Our vagal efficiency is poor, and the vital feedback mechanisms that regulate our heart, lungs, and gut become dampened. Issues such as anxiety, depression, loneliness, and disturbing thoughts may arise. In severe cases, this dysregulation can escalate to self-harm and suicidal thoughts and actions.

An astonishing aspect of Ruth's story is that her hallucinations stopped after just 30 minutes of listening to SSP Core. This outcome prompts curiosity about the underlying mechanisms at play in complex cases like this. Preliminary research suggests a link between low vagal efficiency and intrusive thoughts, including perseverative thinking and hearing voices, which can be considered a form of intrusive thought.[4] Low vagal efficiency is also associated with psychological distress and chronic inflammation. Research indicates that stimulating the vagus nerve may help reduce inflammation and alleviate symptoms.[5]

Implications for Daily Life

Severe dysregulation of the nervous system can lead to profound physical and mental consequences, affecting bodily functions and mental well-being, often manifesting as stress, anxiety, and physical ailments. These ongoing challenges can leave individuals and their caregivers feeling powerless and desperate.

---

* Polyvagal Insight 7: The ANS Can Be Retuned to Prioritize Connection and Well-Being

After exploring numerous treatments for symptoms without relief, many people find themselves depleted of energy, resources, and hope. This frustration is understandable but can distract from addressing the root cause of their issues.

Given the central role of the ANS in mental and physical health, addressing dysregulation is essential for healing. Focusing on stabilizing the ANS can facilitate greater regulation. By raising awareness of how physiological states influence sensations, thoughts, emotions, and behaviors and incorporating activities that promote regulation, nervous system chaos can be reduced, balance can be restored, and health and wellness can gradually be achieved.

Chapter 9

Uwase's Recovery from Disabling Dissociation

Case Overview

SSP PROVIDER: Jennifer (Jenny) Spencer, PhD, HSPP, owner of Spencer Psychology. Website: spencerpsychology.com/jennifer -spencer/

CLINICAL DISCIPLINE: Psychologist and research associate with the Kinsey Institute Traumatic Stress Research Consortium, Indiana University

OTHER THERAPEUTIC MODALITIES AND EXPERTISE: Cognitive behavioral therapy (CBT), eye movement desensitization and reprocessing (EMDR), ego state therapy, Somatic Experiencing, and PVT

CLIENT: Uwase (a pseudonym) was born in a war-torn country. Her family fled their home, spent four months in a refugee camp, and immigrated to the US. These deeply traumatic experiences had enduring impacts on her whole family. Uwase struggled in college, had difficulty establishing trust in relationships, and felt she was just "trudging through life." She began working with Jenny when she was in her early 20s.

FEATURES/SYMPTOMS: Lack of focus, depression, paranoia, suicidal thoughts, nightmares, anxiety, chronic pain, and severe dissociation. She was diagnosed with post-traumatic stress disorder (PTSD) with dissociative features.

AUTONOMIC TENDENCY: The cyclic defense loop, an oscillation between sympathetic and dorsal vagal states

ASSESSMENTS: Body Perception Questionnaire Autonomic Symptoms scale (BPQ20-ANS), PTSD Checklist for DSM-5 (PCL-5), and the Minnesota Multiphasic Personality Inventory-2 (MMPI-2)

Client Description

Uwase and her family escaped the terrors of war and resettled in the US when she was a toddler, having endured numerous harrowing experiences. During the initial stages of increasing conflicts in their area, her father stood guard outside their home at night with a shotgun to protect them from potential attackers. Later, they faced life-threatening conditions in a refugee camp established to shelter those forcibly displaced by targeted persecution and violence. Uwase couldn't remember anyone in her family ever feeling safe.

Once settled in the US, Uwase spent much of her childhood hiding from her father's emotional, verbal, and physical abuse, and her parents divorced when she was in her early adulthood due to his violence. Although distanced from her family while she was attending college in another town, she visited them on birthdays and holidays. Her mother developed multiple gastrointestinal and several other health concerns that were exacerbated by language barriers and poverty.

Uwase was the only one in her family to leave their hometown and pursue higher education. She sought therapy during college, after struggling with difficulty focusing, suicidal thoughts, nightmares, anxiety, and dissociation. Although she initially denied any trauma history, she occasionally commented, "I sometimes don't feel like I'm alive."

Uwase's early counseling consisted of CBT and positive psychology geared to helping her maintain enough stability to finish college and to address her chronic pain. Her college life was marked by loneliness, relationship failures, and feelings of disconnection from her peers and of being deprived of a normal college experience. She developed sexual issues and severe abdominal pain, which required extensive treatment, physical therapy, medication, and a limited diet. Dissociation was her primary, albeit involuntary, coping mechanism. Her persistence in therapy and in college enabled her to graduate, and she has worked since then with steady employment.

Trauma research using brain scans was still relatively new when Uwase began therapy, and less was known about treating clients with severe early trauma like hers. Therapies used with her included EMDR, ego state therapy, Somatic Experiencing, and polyvagal-informed strategies. EMDR was soon stopped because it caused Uwase to have panic attacks and vivid flashbacks of sexual abuse. At first Uwase couldn't tolerate remembering her sexual abuse, nor articulate a full narrative. Ego state therapy helped by revealing that her panic was her younger parts of self recalling her abuse.

Somatic Experiencing and polyvagal-informed strategies significantly reduced how often Uwase felt overwhelmed and/or disabled by panic attacks, but they only moderately lessened her dissociation.

Continued use of ego state techniques helped clarify Uwase's dissociative episodes by enabling her parts of self to become more distinct. Her youngest parts held memories of her abuse, while an angry teenager, called her Guardian during therapy, fiercely prevented access to her vulnerable toddler selves. She also had an adult Professional part representing her working self that functioned competently in a near-constant dissociated state.

Uwase described her experience of life as her adult self trying to steer a ship while her younger parts tried to forcibly take control of the wheel and drown them all if her abuse was acknowledged. This shed light on how she kept the memories of abuse dissociated from her adult life for adaptive reasons. While she continued to make progress in therapy, she still spent significant periods of time in a dissociated state during which she couldn't feel her body and didn't want to anyway because it was saturated with physical and emotional pain.

SSP Delivery Method

When Jenny asked Uwase to try SSP Core in August 2021 (many years into their work together), Uwase was willing to explore anything that might help.

Within seconds of listening, however, she would have a panic attack or dissociate. She and Jenny developed a routine in which Uwase listened for a few seconds, paused for grounding and support, listened for a few more seconds, and then moved into other modalities for the remainder of her session. Over time she was able to tolerate longer listening intervals.

SSP enabled Uwase to access her dysregulated nervous system without her narrative of abuse triggering immediate dissociation. Her inability to tolerate even mild activation had hindered progress in other treatment approaches. When listening to SSP, however, she could experience small increments of activation and stop the music when needed. This let her learn to regulate herself in a gradual, manageable way that hadn't been possible with other modalities.

As Uwase continued with SSP, she started recognizing signs of dissociation and became better at managing increased stimulation without panicking or shutting down. She still hesitated to do deep work on her abuse, however, fearing that she would become trapped for days, as she sometimes did, in complete shutdown—a "paralyzing darkness"—that made it difficult to move, think, or function.

With time and continued listening, Uwase discovered that her nervous system could handle some distress and recover from it. With Jenny's steadfast co-regulation during therapy, Uwase learned to focus on her body, recognize feelings of activation and shutdown, and calm herself. Gradually, she experienced longer periods without dissociating. She began to trust that she could allow herself to feel without being overwhelmed.

Uwase took seven months to complete the five hours of SSP. Because the input from SSP could be separated from the repressed narrative of abuse that activated her, SSP enabled her to learn emotional regulation.* Her new resilience marked a profound and transformative milestone.

---

* Polyvagal Insight 3: Neuroception Detects Cues of Threat and Safety and Alters Autonomic State

Summary of Provider's Observations about the Client's Response to SSP

After years of consistent but slow progress, within a month after completing SSP Uwase was able to acknowledge her feelings of loneliness and recognize that she needed a new job.* Although she had known intellectually that her work environment was toxic, her dissociation had prevented her from feeling the need for change.

She realized that she had lived for years in the same apartment complex where she had resided during college. She also saw that her reluctance to date and risk emotional distress or heartbreak had denied her the possibility of love.

Driven by her new self-awareness, Uwase mobilized. She found a new job in a different city where she could have a wider social circle. She got a new apartment and began exploring the world of dating, a bold step toward a more connected and fulfilling life.

During Uwase's and Jenny's years of working together before SSP, Uwase had appeared calm and in control even when she wasn't because dissociation was her norm. She relied on her Professional to run her life. Her Professional was successful at work, paid her rent, cooked her meals, fed her pets, and showed up for therapy. But Uwase had no sense of an authentic adult self. Her child parts could wrest control from her Professional unless her Guardian blocked them out.

After SSP, Uwase's Guardian reluctantly allowed the emergence of child parts that held memories of her past traumas. Uwase was strong enough now to endure flashes of memory of sexual abuse. She believed it most likely occurred at the refugee camp when she was a toddler. She remembered how her body felt along with scraps of imagery. As time passed, she began to sense that her body held memories of torture. She also felt that she might never have a complete narrative because she was so young when these things happened. She had substantial hope, however, that she could fully heal without needing to remember every detail.

---

* Polyvagal Insight 1: Autonomic State Functions as an Intervening Variable

Two years after Uwase completed SSP, her panic attacks significantly reduced in frequency and severity. She had entered into a romantic relationship that she later ended due to her boyfriend's infidelity and dishonesty. She had allowed herself to love him, be hurt, and have her adult self set boundaries. While she did dissociate in the early months of the relationship, allowing herself not to feel the mounting effects of his emotional abuse, she did not need to dissociate due to her heartbreak. Instead, she stood up for herself and recognized that she didn't have to allow abuse in her life. She still had work to do in therapy, but after SSP, her capacity had expanded significantly, allowing her to engage in the work in a more effective way.

Assessments

Body Perception Questionnaire and PCL-5 Results

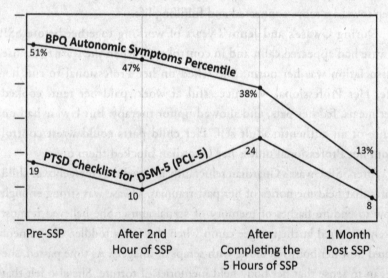

BPQ20-ANS

The BPQ20-ANS measures how often autonomic symptoms are experienced. Autonomic symptoms can be caused by the disruption of typical organ function by chronic threat responses and are more frequently reported in those with a trauma history.[1] Moderate levels of symptoms (e.g., 50th percentile) are associated with sympathetic reactions that are sustained even after the physiological need has passed, while low symptoms are associated with flexible autonomic responses that can engage and return to baseline effectively.[2] As illustrated, Uwase started SSP at a moderate level of symptoms (51st percentile) and over time reduced her scores down to low levels (13th percentile).

PCL-5

Uwase had an 11-point drop from baseline to completion of SSP in her trauma scores, primarily in subscales related to reduced hyperarousal, negative cognitions, and improved mood. This represents a clinically significant change according to the evidence for PCL-5 for DSM-5.[3]

The lowered hyperarousal matched her clinical presentation, as it appeared that activation from hyperarousal in her body was the primary trigger for dissociative episodes and panic attacks.

Uwase had been in treatment for many years before starting SSP, making steady progress on her severe PTSD symptoms. Her initial scores on the PCL were lower than is typical for those diagnosed with PTSD as a result. However, given her severe dissociation and emotional dysregulation, treatment was still ongoing. The dissociation was the primary target at that point in therapy.

There was an interesting increase in symptoms measured by the PCL-5 immediately after SSP completion, while the BPQ showed a steady decrease in autonomic symptoms. This matched her clinical presentation, as she was allowing herself to emotionally experience feelings other than panic or shutdown. As she gained better control over managing her emotional state, her PCL-5 score dropped again. She simply needed to practice allowing feelings, without fearing that her child parts would, as she said, "drown us all."

MMPI-2

Uwase took the MMPI-2 in 2014 and again in 2022 after completing SSP. Concurrent regular therapy, as described above, was also occurring during these years.

In 2014, Uwase's original MMPI-2 scores exhibited a pattern of chronic psychological maladjustment, with high scores on measures of anxiety, depression, trauma, impulse control issues, acting out, substance use, avoidance, denial, and suicidal thoughts. She reported difficulty managing routine affairs and had problems with memory, concentration, and making decisions. Uwase also endorsed feeling immobilized and withdrawn, with no energy. Her original scores noted substantial issues with physical health and numerous somatic concerns.

In 2022, after completing SSP, Uwase's scores were substantially improved, though guarded, with depression, anger, anxiety, and health concerns now in the normal to near-normal ranges.

Summary of Client's Reflections on Their Response to SSP

Uwase experienced SSP as "life changing" and was ever grateful for Jenny's constancy and unwavering support. Two years after Uwase completed the SSP Core, its effects were still apparent. Her improvement was evident in her overall demeanor—she exuded a newfound sense of calmness, connection, and empowerment. Perhaps most significant was her revelation that she had previously lacked a fundamental feeling of safety in her life. She recognized how her new nervous system regulation and sense of safety impacted the quality of her relationships with others and herself, as well as her overall quality of life.*

Uwase's expanded nervous system capacity allowed for many substantial life changes as well as further growth in therapy. For example, she now felt ready to engage in EMDR, another step in her healing journey.

As she continued to integrate and become more embodied, she went through a phase of realizing how deeply she had really struggled. Dissociation had invaded her whole life, numbing her from emotional pain. Sensing her body now required her to accept that terrible experiences had occurred and to stop hiding them from herself. To address her

---

* Polyvagal Insight 8: The ANS Is at the Core of Our Physical and Mental Wellness

painful memories, she continued her individual therapeutic work with Jenny and joined a supportive therapy group.

Thinking back to earlier days, she remembered cycling between irritation, anger, and depression amid the background of constant pain. Her dissociation had been so severe that she had gone through periods when she couldn't move or reach out for support. She'd felt detached, as if she weren't a participant in her own life and was merely watching herself engage in conversations and tasks.

She had much more control of her dissociation now. She could see it as a coping skill. If she were in an intolerable situation, she could "click out," but she could also come back. She saw that dissociation had shielded her from her trauma and helped her to survive. It got her through her teens and twenties so she could grow to be functional despite all the complications that could have derailed her. She could now appreciate her dissociation, recognizing its protective role in her life.

Case Analysis with Dr. Porges

Early in their work together Jenny saw that Uwase's trauma narrative could easily trigger dissociation or a panic attack. When that happened Jenny suggested a walk with Uwase around the building to shift her autonomic state. Being outside together gave Uwase the opportunity for mobilization and co-regulation.* While effective, this carefully attuned work together was a slow process.

SSP Allows a Focus on State Instead of Story

When Uwase and Jenny began using SSP, Uwase was relieved to move her focus away from her "story" and instead concentrate on features of her physiological state. When the SSP music triggered a shift, they would pause the music while the response was still at a low intensity. They would then process the sensations associated with the physiological state without having to deal with her story at the same time. This helped Uwase to become aware that she could experience some dysregulation

---

* Polyvagal Insight 4: The Power of Social Connection and Co-Regulation

and then re-regulate. With this regular and repeated experience with Jenny alongside her, Uwase became better at separating her feelings from her narrative and regulating herself, even when Jenny wasn't around. She learned that her body could handle small levels of distress and recover.*

The filtering in the SSP music sends subconscious signals of safety. However, if someone has a history of trauma, then the signals of safety may be interpreted as signals of threat, triggering a defensive response instead of accessibility. Jenny and Uwase went slowly with SSP, sometimes listening to it only seconds at a time. This approach allowed Uwase to gradually receive signals of safety without experiencing unmanageable distress and to incrementally increase her nervous system flexibility.

SSP is a passive pathway of therapy and is a helpful preparation for other more active therapeutic interventions, which can facilitate further processing and integration. In Uwase's case, SSP allowed her to engage with EMDR, which she hadn't previously been able to do without being emotionally overwhelmed.

SSP Reduced Uwase's Dissociation

Dissociation is an adaptive survival response to intense and overwhelming life-threatening experiences and effectively shuts down conscious awareness, memories, and sensation associated with the event. Dr. Ruth Lanius describes dissociation as "providing an escape where no actual escape is possible. It provides a mental escape from intense experience, from intense emotions, and from intense memories."[4]

Consistent with Dr. Lanius's view, dissociation through the lens of PVT infers an adaptive progressive sequence initially starting with profound immobilization via dorsal vagal pathways, followed by behaviorally freezing as the nervous system adaptively infuses sympathetic tone to maintain posture and consciousness, and finally to dissociative states that, if transitory, minimally compromise autonomic regulation.

While dissociation can serve as a protective shield from the full impact of a traumatic experience, it may lead to a disconnection or detachment

---

* Polyvagal Insight 7: The ANS Can Be Retuned to Prioritize Connection and Well-Being

from one's own thoughts, feelings, identity, or sensations. In Uwase's case, her disconnection was initially so pervasive and debilitating that she would dissociate sometimes for days and lose all sense of time. She felt that she was in a "deep abyss" from which she couldn't even contact Jenny for support. Her dissociation was initially so profound that she was unable to acknowledge or remember her trauma history, which included significant events such as experiencing sexual abuse and witnessing domestic violence in her childhood home.

The work Jenny did with Uwase was instrumental in helping Uwase to understand her own experience of her autonomic states and in learning how to regulate herself. Small experiences of dysregulation and subsequent re-regulation led to being better able to move through the autonomic continuum. SSP played a vital role in this work. It retuned her nervous system.

As Uwase expanded her nervous system capacity and became more resilient, she experienced shorter and less intense periods of dissociation, and she was able to recover from them with fewer residual effects. At times, a moment of dissociation felt like simply a few seconds of daydreaming. As her dissociation episodes shortened and diminished with her increased resilience, she developed more clarity about them. This increased awareness allowed her to monitor her bodily feelings and develop strategies to support her system.[*]

Uwase had experienced horrific early trauma, which led to years of adversity from profound dysregulation and dissociation, yet she managed to find the strength and courage to persevere with therapy to eventually create a connected and capable way to live her life. She has "a kind heart" and is a good friend to others, according to Jenny. Uwase's unwavering commitment to therapy coupled with her luck in finding a skilled, devoted, and consistently co-regulating therapist like Jenny played a crucial role. Now, with less dissociation, Uwase has a new trajectory in life—one that is not limited by the debilitating impact of her trauma.

---

[*] Polyvagal Insight 7: The ANS Can Be Retuned to Prioritize Connection and Well-Being

Implications for Daily Life

Wars and crimes against humanity leave a lasting impact on individuals and their descendants, creating repercussions that span generations. However, even the most severe complex trauma caused by these and other horrific traumatic experiences can be mitigated through the constancy, deep respect, and attentive presence of a highly skilled clinician. Effective therapy, conducted at a pace suited to the individual and facilitated by a clinician who prioritizes relationship, connection, and co-regulation, can make a significant difference. When combined with tools such as SSP, this approach has the potential to reduce dissociation and foster meaningful healing in the aftermath of trauma. This can bring great hope for refugees who have survived war and torture. The benefits are long-lasting and may even prevent the transmission of trauma to the next generation.

Chapter 10

A Family Heals from Shock and Grief

Case Overview

SSP PROVIDER: Ana do Valle, OTR, SEP, anthroposophical counselor, founder of the Soma Healing Center. Website: somahealingcenter.com

CLINICAL DISCIPLINE AND FOCUS: Ana is an occupational therapist, Somatic Experiencing Practitioner, and an anthroposophical counselor who specializes in working with the nervous system and the body/soul/spirit. She created the SEGAN model, a multisensory listening and art-based model for treating children, couples, and adults who present with difficulties in the areas of affect and behavioral regulation.

OTHER THERAPEUTIC MODALITIES AND EXPERTISE: Anthroposophical counseling, sensory processing, Somatic Experiencing, and PVT

CLIENTS: Melanie, her 15-year-old son Clay, and 10-year-old daughter Sophia (all pseudonyms) experienced the sudden death of Greg (their husband and father) at age 48. Four months later, they traveled to spend a week with Ana in Boulder, Colorado, each bringing their individual experience of shock and grief.

FEATURES/SYMPTOMS: In addition to the shock and grief they all experienced, Clay was working on his relational skills, and Sophia had withdrawn from communication and her family had become used to speaking for her. In addition to managing her own grief, Melanie was supporting Clay and Sophia and keeping them unified.

AUTONOMIC TENDENCY: Melanie: dorsal vagal; Clay: oscillating in a cyclic defense loop between the defensive states of sympathetic (with a fight tendency) and dorsal; Sophia: freeze and dorsal vagal

ASSESSMENTS: Beyond Ana's standard intake process and measures, no formal assessments were utilized.

Client Description

Melanie's husband, Greg, died suddenly at age 48 after a COVID illness. She found him early one morning without a pulse in a chair in their bedroom. She called 911, the emergency phone number, and the responder talked her through administering cardiopulmonary resuscitation to Greg. Meanwhile, sirens approached their home, and multiple paramedics entered the house with their loud boots and voices. Melanie watched as they tried in vain to resuscitate him. Clay and Sophia were awakened by the commotion and learned of their father's death amid this chaos. They were all still in a state of shock four months later when they arrived in Boulder for their work with Ana.

Their family was tightly knit and deeply connected. Melanie had been homeschooling the children since before their father's death to best support their unique needs and aspirations. Among their goals were helping Sophia find her voice and guiding Clay to overcome his anger and isolation.

Each of them was responding to Greg's death according to their autonomic tendencies: Melanie had lost hope for the future and was tearful and worried about her children; Clay was overwhelmed with anger; and Sophia's terror would surface at times, leaving her unable to speak.

Melanie wanted to heal herself and her children and restore normalcy for them but recognized that she needed help to do so. She chose to work with Ana because of her SEGAN model, a bottom-up approach to SSP delivery with five phases that correspond to the five hours of SSP listening. Incorporating sensation, emotion, gesture, action, and narrative, Ana invites imagination, inspiration, and intuition to strengthen the capacity for being present with ourselves and each other.

SSP Delivery Method

Melanie, Clay, and Sophia each listened to a full hour of SSP Core with Ana each day outdoors on a farm with horses, donkeys, cats, and chickens. Above them, hawks and eagles soared across the wide-open sky. The family's intentions for the week were to heal their grief, find movement out of their place of hopelessness and sadness, and support each other.

They spent the entire week together, with Ana gently guiding them to explore nature, read stories, create art, and work with horses in addition to their SSP listening. One of the books they read together was about a wounded owl who found safety through connection with others and learned that love endures despite adverse life events. The owl, symbolizing life, death, and rebirth, became significant to them when all three spotted one on their first day. Since then, owls have held great importance for the family.

Every day, along with their SSP sessions, Ana encouraged creative activities such as writing poems, painting with watercolors, and sculpting with clay. Watercolors helped them explore emotions through colors, while clay fostered willpower. Because shock often induces a cold sensation and can lead to dissociation, they also warmed beeswax in their hands to counteract the cold and shock.

Ana provided no specific instructions on what to create, allowing experiences and emotions to surface naturally in their artwork. Clay crafted tools like swords, arrowheads, and spears, reflecting his inner "warrior" and survivor spirit. Meanwhile, Sophia made delicate wool-felted animals and hearts expressing her gentle nature.

Ana utilized the creative process to reintroduce movement and rhythm into their daily lives, opening sensory channels for healing and fostering creation and transformation. She invited Melanie, Clay, and Sophia to sculpt archetypal characters in beeswax to craft a family fairytale. Clay made a blue snake, Sophia created a broken pink heart patched back together, and Melanie's character wore a black superhero cape. Together, they improvised a tale that began with a fire and ended with each of them gaining superpowers, symbolizing their journey toward hope and courage. Creating this story together helped the family face their trauma, providing grounding, orientation, and resilience in the face of their tragedy. The fairytale allowed each family member to play an active role in their healing process.

Another profound experience was spending time with horses where the effects of SSP were particularly powerful. Horses, known for their sensitivity, helped open the family's sensory channels, fostering greater embodiment, coherence, and healing. The rhythmic breathing of the horses regulated the family's own breathing. As their exhales lengthened and their shoulders relaxed, Ana noticed a stronger connection forming among the three of them. Grief can be bound with the breath, and the horses were instrumental in helping reset the rhythm of their breathing. The horses responded to this shift as well, periodically offering happy, pulsed snorts that made everyone laugh.* This allowed for even deeper breathing and the release of buried memories.

Riding one of the horses, a wild mustang, further enhanced their sense of groundedness, giving them the experience of being one with the horse and its movement. This supported their ability to stay present in their bodies, balanced and aligned, as they moved through space and time.

On the final day, Melanie, Clay, and Sophia envisioned their future together as a family and how they wanted to support each other moving forward. They could now picture a life for themselves without Greg. They completed their experience with a healing ceremony using baby's

---

* Polyvagal Insight 4: The Power of Social Connection and Co-Regulation

breath flowers, which are commonly associated with new beginnings. They tapped the flowers on their skin to bring more of their awareness into the present moment. Then they released the baby's breath into the cold waters of the flowing river to symbolize the letting go of a tragic moment that would no longer prevent them from embracing life.

Summary of Provider's Observations about the Clients' Response to SSP

Every activity during the family's retreat was chosen to help integrate their hearts and minds, enabling them to articulate their sensations and emotions within a coherent narrative. This approach fostered a sense of wholeness and presence among them. Engaging in multisensory activities such as outdoor experiences, working with beeswax, and interacting with horses helped them soften their thinking processes and increased their adaptability. The rhythmic patterns of the SSP music and the cues of safety in the filtering influenced their breathing, enhanced their capacity to feel, and facilitated their personal and collective healing journey. Throughout each day of SSP delivery, Melanie, Clay, and Sophia made steady progress in their individual healing processes.

Several factors contributed to the remarkable healing experienced by this family in a short period: the immersive nature of the experience, extended time spent together, separation from their daily routines, immersion in nature, physical movement, and artistic engagement. The containment and retuning of the ANS provided by SSP, combined with activities involving proprioceptive, vestibular, tactile, and visual sensory inputs, heightened their awareness of the present moment. Thus, the family's participation in both SSP and diverse outdoor activities created a mosaic of healing and renewed hope, benefitting each member individually and strengthening their familial bonds.

Melanie transitioned from feeling hopeless about the future to feeling internally strong and confident, anchored by her children and open to exploring new ways to support herself upon returning home.

Clay's anger diminished, giving way to a calmer demeanor and a more supportive attitude toward his mother and sister. Back home, he took on cooking duties for the family. While he still felt a responsibility to protect them, he began to focus less on his "warrior" persona and started engaging more playfully with their cats, even mimicking the flapping wings of the blue heron he had enjoyed at the farm, reflecting a new lighter side of himself.

Sophia grew less fearful and embraced joy more readily. Previously reliant on Melanie and Clay to speak for her in new situations, she found herself needing their assistance less. Sophia started participating in activities at the recreation center, including gymnastics, and socializing with peers her age. This newfound engagement helped her shift out of a shutdown state and into a more socially connected ventral vagal state.

Each family member navigated their dissociative states uniquely, rediscovering their zest for life. Their stuckness, grief, and shock were gradually replaced by resilience, possibility, and hope. As they learned to be present with each other and express their emotions openly, their bond deepened, fostering ongoing healing that could continue, perhaps for years. They now move forward with a renewed sense of purpose and direction.

Summary of Clients' Reflections on Their Responses to SSP

Melanie, Clay, and Sophia were worried about each other after Greg's death but could not create forward movement, release their pain, or freely express themselves. However, six weeks after SSP and Ana's SEGAN process, each of them had changed in individual ways.

Melanie regained her grounding, which enabled her to attend to the numerous responsibilities that arose after Greg's passing. Instead of drowning in overwhelm, grief, and shock, she could breathe again, feel peace, and draw strength from within. She reflected, "I honestly don't know how I would have coped without SSP."

Four months after the family's healing retreat, Ana followed up with them to check on their progress. Melanie shared, "I'm prioritizing my emotions more now. I've been active and making more time for movement." She was undergoing EMDR therapy to manage anxiety and flashbacks. She had joined a grief support group where she found solace in reading several books like *Healing After Loss* by Martha W. Hickman, *It's OK That You're Not OK* by Megan Devine, *After Your Person Dies* by Linda Shanti McCabe, and *The Grieving Brain* by Mary-Frances O'Connor.

Melanie now grasped the relationship between movement, breath, and grief. Understanding how movement could enhance vagal tone, influence brain chemistry, and support regulation, she set a goal to engage in physical activity for one to one and a half hours every day. Her favorite activities were hula hoop (she chuckled as she mentioned this), racquetball, and tai chi. She also found community in her yoga class at the local recreation center where Sophia often joined her.*

Melanie expressed that she was no longer drowning in sadness and remarked, "I can notice when I'm starting to feel overwhelmed and I can handle it."

The family was connecting regularly, particularly at bedtime when they had long discussions about what was going on with each of them. They were all disappointed that it was too cold to spend as much time outdoors as they liked, especially because they remembered how much they enjoyed that with Ana. The three of them were talking about moving to California where they had friends and the weather was better. Sophia loved the ocean, and Clay would be able to integrate better into the community there.

Clay reported that he gained some peace and quiet from SSP. He felt that when he was in Boulder, he had a place where he could relax. When asked what has lasted since then, he answered, "A peaceful mind." SSP helped him release his racing thoughts and worries, allowing him to focus on his sensations and feelings. He felt he was doing much better with his emotions—he could pause and recognize what he was feeling whereas before he couldn't. He still got angry, but now he could notice it and stay more present.†

---

* Polyvagal Insight 4: The Power of Social Connection and Co-Regulation

† Polyvagal Insight 1: Autonomic State Functions as an Intervening Variable

Sophia's dominant reaction to her father's death had been intense fear. Four months later, she reported that she felt "a lot calmer and more energized" and that she could "listen better." After waking up to the sounds of sirens and first responders in her home attempting to revive her father, she hadn't been able to listen very well or hear people clearly, but her hearing was better now.* Listening to SSP had allowed her association with sound to reset. She had even joined a children's choir and sang with them after school. At the recreation center where she went regularly by herself, she jumped rope and played basketball and Ping-Pong. Sometimes, she, Clay, and her mother went together. She mentioned feeling more courageous now and, in general, she experiences increased feelings of happiness, energy, and calmness.†

Melanie acknowledged that each one of them had made significant progress, emphasized that there was still more work ahead, and reassured them by saying, "It's OK that we are not OK."

Case Analysis with Dr. Porges

Grieving the loss of a loved one is a unique type of trauma in which the infliction of the traumatic event is from someone you love and are connected to but who is no longer there to comfort you. Thrust suddenly into a new reality, Melanie and her children found themselves grappling with intense emotions and bodily reactions. The experience of Greg's unexpected death violated their sense of expectancy, of protection, and of trust. Ultimately, there was also a sense of abandonment. Greg had left them. Although he wasn't at fault, the family had no warning or preparation for the possibility that he might die. This is very confusing to the nervous system.

Each member of the family was in a state of shock and expressed different presentations of a defensive physiology. When the body perceives

---

* Polyvagal Insight 6: Autonomic State, Vocal Intonation, and Middle Ear Muscle Regulation Mutually Influence Each Other

† Polyvagal Insight 7: The ANS Can Be Retuned to Prioritize Connection and Well-Being

an extreme threat, it responds by either intensifying or reducing the volume of emotions, sensations, behavior, and thinking.*

Additionally, the emotions and states experienced by one person have the potential to permeate and influence those around them.† The experience of grieving is deeply physiological and affects the whole body. It's not a psychological phenomenon that we have control over.

Top-down processes can be unhelpful in recovering from grief. In fact, they may even make things worse. Rumination and perseverative thinking often occur in individuals experiencing a sudden and overwhelming wave of grief. They can engage in "what if" thinking that imagines, unhelpfully, how the outcome of the source of their grief could have been different. This is distracting and interferes with life and relationships. And yet, it is common for a nervous system stuck in a state of threat to have less flexibility and to become trapped by detrimental thoughts. These thoughts can lead to a more defensive state and a downward spiral.

A more effective way forward is to focus on a somatic and physiological approach rather than a purely cognitive one. That said, grief is a process, not a state. Again and again, our body has to detect safety, understanding, and support. Cooperation, trust, and love become possible again when we are in supportive environments where we can let go of our defenses. Nature is very helpful in this regard as it reconnects us with the essence of life and living. Ana intuitively understood that bringing the family to the farm would help them feel less threatened and be able to give up their defensiveness. It was also helpful for them to be away from home where reminders of what had happened, all that needed to be done, and what would happen next were everywhere. Stepping out of their normal life to be together in nature gave them the capacity to be themselves, to be synergistic together, and to become a tighter family unit.

---

* Polyvagal Insight 1: Autonomic State Functions as an Intervening Variable

† Polyvagal Insight 3: Neuroception Detects Cues of Threat and Safety and Alters Autonomic State

Giving Up Defenses

Ana believed that they could find their warmth and connection again in a more safe and hopeful way. She understood that it was important for them to *feel* again and to reembrace life. This required them to trust and feel safe enough to go along with the journey. Being at the farm, guided by Ana's intuition and immersed in their connection with each other and nature, helped ground them and warm them to their surroundings, waking up their senses. This environment provided valuable resources to their nervous systems, supporting their healing process.

When we're under threat, our senses operate differently. Primed for cues of danger, our neuroception causes us to perceive almost all stimuli as potentially harmful. However, in a safe environment where we can lower our defenses, our neuroception shifts from a focus on danger and can instead be driven by curiosity. This was the case for Melanie, Clay, and Sophia. Supported by Ana's intuitive guidance, wisdom, and experience in somatic and spiritual practices, they were invited into a space of healing. Once they could savor the experiences of the natural beauty, connection, and creative expression, their sensory pathways became a source of nourishment.[*]

Ana described that "because thinking is influenced by new perceptions, there was a softening in their thinking that also freed their will to move toward life again." In polyvagal terms, this can be reframed as "When we relinquish defenses, curiosity emerges, leading to optimism."

Shifts into defensive states are not inherently negative, but it can be challenging if we are unaware of these changes and their impact on us. Being aware allows us to see how our state colors our perspective of the world. We can continue being driven by reactivity, and our state changes, or we can recognize our autonomic shifts and tendencies and respond with greater mindfulness. In essence, this encapsulates the goal of all therapy: to reembody oneself and recognize that a loving, trusting life necessitates letting go of defenses and cultivating self-awareness. SSP supports this transformative process by retuning the nervous system toward safety.

---

[*] Polyvagal Insight 7: The ANS Can Be Retuned to Prioritize Connection and Well-Being

Trust and Connection

Our physiology is naturally designed to connect and co-regulate. Our relationships play a vital role in helping us feel safe after encountering perceived threats. But paradoxically, when we encounter a threat, we may retreat from those relationships. People who are grieving have a physiology of threat and vulnerability. Having a relationship with someone who can validate their experience will give much-needed signals of trust and safety that will allow them to let down their defensiveness. Trusting relationships help to facilitate healing.[*]

Ana cultivated a deep sense of trust with Melanie, Clay, and Sophia, fostering a strong and supportive relationship. She offered many experiences to help them to move out of their threat states. Her own presence and SSP both sent signals of safety that were "enablers" of therapy. This helped the family to become more aware of their bodily reactions and to become more embodied and not locked in physiological states of threat. In addition, SSP, nature, wildlife, watercolors, sculpting with clay and beeswax, poetry, family stories, and their closing ritual were all neural exercises for coming back to safety.

Since returning to their life, social engagement has been important to all of them. The whole family has good social support. Each child has a good friend and activities to be together with other people. Melanie, too, has supportive friends and family checking in on her. She also takes regular salt baths, reads, does yoga, and is in a grief support group and regular therapy. Their three friendly family cats add to the co-regulation in their life.

Rituals

Every culture has a ritual around the death of a loved one. Rituals provide a safe container for the expression and release of intense emotions. Melanie, Clay, and Sophia felt that the closing ceremony at the farm where they threw baby's breath flowers into the river was more personal and maybe more healing than Greg's funeral service.

---

[*] Polyvagal Insight 4: The Power of Social Connection and Co-Regulation

Clay expressed feeling "lighter." He was able to release his anger and become more grounded in his body during that experience. It marked a meaningful culmination of their time together, fostering further healing and strengthening their bond as a new family unit. It appeared to reinforce their commitment to supporting each other with increased tenderness.

Since returning home, they have gravitated toward some rituals of their own making. One involves spending time together before sleep, when they each share details about their day, thoughts, and feelings. This nightly routine provides a regular chance to co-regulate and is a significant cue of safety for their nervous systems. They have also returned to Pizza Fridays, a tradition that started when Greg was alive. It's a predictable part of their week they all look forward to. Additionally, eating together holds significance as it enhances social engagement. Ingestion and social engagement are connected within the same neural circuit, reinforcing one another. As a ritual, sharing a meal has positive consequences for our neurobiology.

Implications for Daily Life

Grief is a process, not a state. By ensuring continued access to the SES through nervous system regulation, one may navigate the grieving process more effectively. Rituals, trust, interpersonal connections, engagement with nature, artistic expressions, and ventral vagal exercises send signals of safety to our body and promote nervous system flexibility. This fosters resilience and facilitates the healing journey.

Chapter 11

Shifting from Perfectionism to Being "Perfectly Imperfect"

Case Overview

> **SSP PROVIDER:** Michael Allison, performance coach, developer of The Play Zone, a science-based approach to optimize resilience and performance in sport and life. Website: theplayzone.com
>
> **CLINICAL DISCIPLINE:** Michael is a performance and wellness coach working with executives, performers, creatives, and athletes using PVT to improve resilience, performance, and enjoyment in their work and play.
>
> **OTHER THERAPEUTIC MODALITIES AND EXPERTISE:** Movement, breath, balance, and PVT
>
> **CLIENT:** Todd, a thoughtful and high-achieving individual in his 60s, excels in various domains—he's a respected lawyer, a top tennis player in his age group, and an accomplished classical pianist. He had been working with Michael on his overall health and performance in tennis, which, in turn, influenced his piano playing and his legal work. SSP was introduced to address his sleep issues.
>
> **FEATURES/SYMPTOMS:** Perfectionism; maintaining high standards in each of the three performance domains of his life: his profession, sport, and music; and poor sleep

AUTONOMIC TENDENCY: Sympathetic activation was Todd's go-to strategy in facing challenges, but this interrupted his sleep.

ASSESSMENTS: Beyond Michael's standard intake process and measures, no formal assessments were utilized.

Client Description

As a trial lawyer, Todd's work required months of meticulous preparation for a case. Every detail had to be at his fingertips when he presented his client's experience and perspective in court, the high-stakes culmination of his comprehensive planning. This same attention to detail and pursuit of excellence permeated the other passions in Todd's life: classical piano and tennis.

Michael had been friends with Todd and had worked with him as his performance coach for nearly 14 years. Michael uses PVT to help his clients recognize their adaptive, reflexive, and predictable bodily reactions to both safety and challenge. He teaches them to unlock their full potential through their physiology by meeting themselves where they are, moment to moment, without shame, blame, or judgment. His clients learn to sense how their bodily state is the source of every component of their performance, including reaction time, creativity, concentration, problem-solving, and feelings of confidence. Clients come to accept that their performance can fluctuate at any time, and to maintain excellence, they must appreciate the factors that are beneath their conscious control that functionally promote or interrupt performance.

Todd incorporated these ideas into his tennis game by focusing his awareness on his physiological states. This enabled him to deliberately shift his breathing depth and pace and reduce muscle tension in his face, neck, shoulders, hands, and belly while playing. He shifted his attention away from the threat of the competition as well as his own inner stories of "not being good enough." Instead, he directed his mind toward who and what was safe, comforting, and reassuring. This allowed him to sense that time seemed to slow "up," enabling him to see key opportunities in the game. He was fascinated by the differences a polyvagal approach made and was pleased it not only enhanced his performance and enjoyment of tennis but other areas of his life as well.

The next area to address was Todd's sleep. His workload, diligence, and the natural processes of aging had worsened his sleep over time. He would awaken in the middle of the night with racing thoughts and be unable to go back to sleep for hours. This was the primary reason for incorporating SSP.

SSP Delivery Method

Michael and Todd had a longstanding relationship built on trust and developed through extensive polyvagal psychoeducation and a clear understanding of how Todd responded to various stresses and state shifts. This strong foundation of safety and communication allowed for the introduction of SSP. Todd would primarily use SSP independently at home, with regular check-ins with Michael to discuss his experiences, knowing Michael was always available by phone if needed. Before his first solo session, they did 10 minutes of SSP listening together so Michael could observe Todd's initial reaction to the filtered music. Todd responded positively during this initial session.

Todd completed his first round of SSP Core in March 2021 by listening in 30-minute sessions on his own. During quiet time in the early evenings, he would sit comfortably on his living room sofa, his back facing the wall. His strong self-regulatory skills, coupled with having Michael just a phone call away, made his listening comfortable. He texted Michael when he started each session and again afterward with notes about what he had experienced including any bodily sensations, emotions, or thoughts that emerged spontaneously. Michael encouraged Todd to shift his attention between the music, his breathing, and bodily sensations.

After completing the five-hour protocol, Todd listened daily over the following two weeks to 30 minutes of either SSP Balance or SSP Connect.

In July of 2021, hoping for further retuning of his ANS, he repeated the full five-hour SSP Core protocol on his own with 30-minute sessions, along with daily check-ins with Michael. He also repeated Hours 3, 4, and 5, turning his listening into an eight-hour protocol.

In September 2021, Todd began using the SSP Core Hours 3, 4, or 5 and SSP Balance intermittently, on an "as needed" basis for state regulation, primarily just before bedtime for 10–20 minutes while lying in bed.

In September 2022, Todd completed SSP Core again, listening 30 minutes per day with daily check-ins. Following this, he continued using SSP Core Hours 3, 4, or 5 on an "as needed" basis for state regulation.

By May of 2023, Todd completed nearly 80 hours of listening time spread across 277 individual sessions, alternating between SSP Core and SSP Balance.

Summary of Provider's Observations about the Client's Response to SSP

Todd's experience with SSP yielded far more than improved sleep, his initial goal. He was already reaping benefits from employing a polyvagal lens in the competitive areas of his life. Now, SSP seemed to enhance the fluidity in his nervous system, with small changes gradually accumulating into larger improvements that enhanced his overall quality of life.[*]

All of these changes stemmed from one fundamental shift: he transitioned from perfectionism to ease. He still had high standards, but his attitude toward them relaxed enough to generate beneficial changes in his thoughts, feelings, and behaviors. More than a mindset, this progress was grounded in his body's improved autonomic regulation, which supported a more functional SES.

Relaxed Expectations of Himself and Others

Todd noticed a shift in how he perceived his performance. During a National Tennis Rating Program age division tennis tournament, he competed against a top player and didn't win, but his reaction was different from previous losses. This time, he recognized that he had learned a great deal and acknowledged that he had performed well against a strong opponent.[†]

---

[*] Polyvagal Insight 7: The ANS Can Be Retuned to Prioritize Connection and Well-Being

[†] Polyvagal Insight 1: Autonomic State Functions as an Intervening Variable

Afterward, he picked up lunch from a local take-out restaurant and noticed they had run out of napkins. Previously, he might have been irritated and questioned what had caused such inefficiency. He might even have had a physical reaction and constructed a narrative about the unacceptability of such mistakes. But not this time. Instead, he laughed, recognizing the futility of reacting in that way.

Being in the Play Zone

Perfectionism can stifle creativity and fluidity. But by adopting a more ease-based approach, Todd started tapping into a state of effortless concentration and optimal performance. His blended state of ventral and sympathetic inched more toward ventral with his vagal brake applied a little more than previously. He experienced increased agility in tennis and reported a sensation of time slowing during some points as he was completely absorbed in the game. His total immersion gave him more time to strategize and easily meet the ball and led to greater enjoyment.

Similar changes were evident in Todd's music. He noticed he was more relaxed and less focused on the technical aspects of a piece. He felt freer while playing. Along with his solid technical proficiency, he now sensed that he was playing with more emotion. His playing sounded better, and he enjoyed letting the music sound "pretty." His wife, an accomplished violinist, pianist, and music teacher, agreed that his playing had improved noticeably; it was "more nuanced and beautiful."

Relationships

Todd also developed a greater openness to engaging in conversations that involved genuine feelings. Through his polyvagal lens and expanded nervous system capacity, he consistently explored what was "underneath the behavior" of others.* This shift toward curiosity made him feel less judgmental, more patient, and kinder toward both others and himself. It also allowed him to "see, hear, and feel the common core of humanity in himself and others."

---

* Polyvagal Insight 2: Autonomic States Bias Our Feelings, Thoughts, and Behaviors

Recovery from Performance Anxiety

As a teen, Todd had played a piece of music by memory for a recital in front of a large group, including friends, parents, and other students. Early in his performance, he made a mistake, stopped, and started over from the beginning. He felt tremendous shame, and after finishing the piece, he quickly left the stage and hid in a back room instead of rejoining the audience. He became afraid of playing from memory in front of others and was even uncomfortable watching other professional musicians performing. The humiliation he experienced was so profound that he avoided putting himself in a similar situation for more than 50 years.

Yet, after his extensive use of SSP, Todd chose to perform Chopin's Etude Op. 10, No. 3 from memory at a recital. He now understood his fear and how his body reflexively responded to the pressure of performing.* He became less critical of himself for experiencing a range of emotions. Most importantly, he let go of the need to be perfect and could drop into the experience of listening, feeling, and being present with the music as it flowed from within him.

Still, it wasn't at all comfortable or easy. At the start of the piece, he struggled with some mistakes, but he stayed with it, letting go of the imperfections. As his wife later described, "He didn't stop, and he ran through the minefield." Gradually, he started to relax, finishing the piece while enjoying the experience and feeling confidently anchored in his play zone.

His performance wasn't perfect, but Todd was happy he did it. He felt good about himself. He had learned that he didn't have to make his nervous feelings go away. Instead, he could respect and accept those feelings as part of being human, relating to his imperfections as being "perfectly imperfect." This was an entirely different and fulfilling internal experience for Todd.

Replacing Perfectionism with Ease

Many clients seeking to improve performance are already highly competent. Perfectionism is abundant among successful people and in our

---

* Polyvagal Insight 3: Neuroception Detects Cues of Threat and Safety and Alters Autonomic State

culture. Striving for excellence is considered a positive trait, but it can be harmful too if it creates rigidity and too much sympathetic energy. Michael observed that SSP "seems to help soften the inner critic and help the body to trust that it's actually safe to feel safe."

Summary of Client's Reflections on Their Response to SSP

SSP had an immediate effect on the quality of Todd's sleep and dream life from his first session of listening. His dreams became and remained more vivid, which he found wonderful. His best sleep tended to come after a booster session of SSP Core, and good sleep enhanced all aspects of his health and life.

Todd sensed that SSP helped his body become more relaxed. His calmness and sense that "everything is fine and will be fine" welcomed dreams. Even if his dream content was unsettling, his body allowed him to remain asleep and see the dream to its conclusion. This had rarely occurred pre-SSP.

Todd's new polyvagal lens and retuned ANS allowed him to understand both his own and other people's behaviors and perspectives in a different way. Seeing the world in this new way became a subconscious habit that enhanced his interpersonal relationships.

Todd often worked closely with clients during challenging times. His keen ability to discern whether they felt safe and resilient or threatened and overwhelmed provided valuable guidance. For example, when a client felt a fair settlement offer was too low, Todd remained calm and patient, using effective timing and approach to help them reach an agreement.

Soon after listening to SSP, Todd sensed greater calm and fluidity in his tennis game. Many describe tennis as a mental game, but Todd now found it to be a distillation of PVT. In tennis, as in life, competition, evaluation, and feelings of isolation are signals of threat to the nervous system. Appreciating this changed how Todd approached playing the game and how he viewed professional tennis.

Todd's new ease opened doors to new opportunities and enjoyment. The effects of his SSP experience and a polyvagal approach to all aspects of his life were cumulative. His ability to recognize his states and shift out of a defensive state were transferable skills that carried over from one domain to another and supported everything he did.*

Overall, Todd expressed that SSP and PVT benefitted him even when he wasn't actively using them because he knew they were available if he needed them. He's not sure where one started and the other ended, but both had transformed him.

Case Analysis with Dr. Porges

This case illuminates how incremental increases in the flexibility of the nervous system can enhance performance from an already high level and improve our lived experience. We see an impact in all domains of Todd's life resulting from a softening around the edges and a dropping of his defenses. The body needs to learn to lower its defenses in order to achieve safety and relaxation. This is the goal of therapy and coaching. When we're defensive, we lose access to clear thinking and discernment. When we're unsafe, our ANS reflexively prioritizes immediate threats, whether they are life-threatening or related to a work deadline.

In Todd's case, the cues of threat from his work and his high-performance standards triggered unconscious defenses, leading to rigidity that impacted various aspects of his life. Through his work with Michael and SSP, which provides unambiguous signals of safety to the nervous system, Todd developed more tolerance toward himself and the world. This led to greater flexibility, enjoyment, and ease.

Leveraging the Defensiveness of Perfectionism

From a polyvagal perspective, one's perfectionism can be linked to either or both defensive states: the activated sympathetic state for performance energy or the immobilized dorsal vagal state if shame, lack of confidence, or obsessive thoughts are involved. Todd's tended to lean toward the sympathetic fight state. His body mobilized with heightened arousal to focus on achievement and avoid mistakes.

---

* Polyvagal Insight 7: The ANS Can Be Retuned to Prioritize Connection and Well-Being

Todd loved to compete. He described his drive as an intense effort to do his best, meet challenges, and win. Even if he lost, he still loved competition because he saw it as the chance to elevate his own performance and challenge himself. In the courtroom, he needed to win for his client, which required preparation, sensitivity, and judgment in his tactics. On the tennis court, he was drawn to high athleticism and strategy. In his classical piano playing, he practiced by immersing himself in the music to achieve both the technical elements and the composer's intended interpretation. His sympathetic nervous system provided the mobilization to do these things.

If Todd's goals relied solely on mobilizing his sympathetic nervous system, his results would have been limited. Intensity is necessary, but so are flexibility, nuance, and artistry. These creative aspects become available only when some ventral vagal regulation is alongside sympathetic activation.

Engaging and releasing the vagal brake allows for movement along the continuum between ventral and sympathetic responses. Shifting between these two primary states is more subtle than binary. As the vagal brake is engaged, our responses move toward ventral, and our defenses are reduced. As the brake is released (due to a neuroception of threat), more sympathetic activation is enabled.

The continuum between the ventral and sympathetic responses is individual and situational, but it may look something like this:

When leaning toward a ventral vagal state, one tends to be more relaxed and connected, which can lead to better performance. Consider

The Continuum Between Ventral and Sympathetic Responses

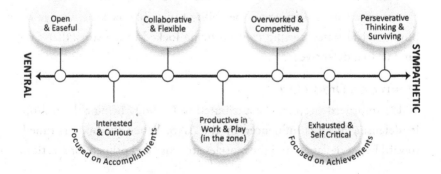

basketball, where free throws are always shot on the exhale. In public speaking, using extended phrases of speech slows the delivery and relaxes the speaker. Solving problems with a relaxed mindset, rather than under the pressure of stress or urgency, often leads to better outcomes. Increased vagal efficiency helps one to finesse the amount of activation needed for the just-right contributions of ventral and sympathetic influence.

Improved Vagal Efficiency May Reduce Obsessive Thinking

Higher vagal efficiency (VE) improves the ability to drop one's defenses. VE is a specific measure of the robustness of the vagal brake inferred from the relationship between heart rate variability (HRV) and heart rate. It indicates more efficient regulation of heart rate and reflects one's ability to respond effectively to stressors and to maintain homeostasis. Higher VE is associated with better access to the ease and sociality of the SES.

Higher VE is also correlated with reduced obsessive thoughts. This relationship was verified in research using fMRI (functional magnetic resonance imaging) to assess activation of the brain's salience network in individuals with high and low vagal efficiency.[1] The salience network is involved in detecting and assessing the importance of sensory inputs, emotional cues, social signals, and events in our environment. The study found that higher VE was associated with more consistent and reliable connection within the salience network. This consistent pattern of activity and connectivity would lead to reduced rumination and perseverative thoughts.

This makes intuitive sense. As Michael describes, "Greater vagal efficiency enhances resilience and the ability to flexibly navigate a range of physiological states, freeing us from being locked into a story that confines us to a defensive state."

Sleep and Dreaming

Todd's improved sleep can be attributed to his body being able to drop its defenses. Sleep is influenced by the ANS. When the body is tuned toward hypervigilance, and the muscles are tense and primed for reaction, sleep becomes elusive because the body is prioritizing defense.* As well as being hard to fall asleep, it is also harder to stay asleep. The ability to relax without any vigilance is the definition of feeling safe enough to be in one's body and to allow the ANS to do one of the things it's meant to do: foster rest and restorative sleep.

Elements of our culture, however, offer enticing distractions that can influence and change us. We minimize the times when we feel safe enough to switch off and just relax. Instead, we are distracted by televisions, computer screens, and cell phones before bed, preventing us from calming down to prepare for a restful sleep.

Our deep stages of sleep are a time of true vulnerability, when our heartbeat and breathing slow to their lowest levels. Our muscles relax, and our ability to monitor the environment is reduced. We are slow in responding once awakened. During REM sleep when most of our dreaming occurs, we experience a kind of paralysis that protects us from acting out our dreams. For Todd, the cues of safety embedded in the filtered music (which he sometimes listened to before bed) enabled his body to move into a state of relaxation, and better sleep was a byproduct.

Todd is now even able to sleep through uncomfortable dreams with ease. He's interested in what his brain is constructing, and he's curious about what it means and how it will play out. This curiosity reflects Todd's new flexibility and increased capacity. His previous tendency was to create negative narratives, but he allows those feelings to play out rather than acting immediately. For Todd, staying asleep through an unsettling dream represents his ability to "let it play out." By creating space between his feelings and actions, both in his waking life and his dreams, he's reinforcing his ability to respond with greater composure.†

---

* Polyvagal Insight 8: The ANS Is at the Core of Our Physical and Mental Wellness

† Polyvagal Insight 1: Autonomic State Functions as an Intervening Variable

Supporting the Effectiveness of SSP

A powerful input to the experience of SSP is the trust and co-regulation between the provider and client.* Sociality and relationships are powerful neuromodulators. Mutual respect, shared interests, and a sense of fun are immediately apparent in Michael and Todd's friendship. Todd is understood and seen by Michael. Additionally, Todd has many other supportive and predictable relationships in his life that contribute to his well-being.

Implications for Daily Life

At our core, we all yearn for an environment where we can truly be ourselves, celebrating our unique talents, creativity, and compassion. When we lack a sense of safety, however, these qualities become stifled, and we can't flourish to our full potential. Our pursuit of perfection often hampers our efforts, paradoxically diminishing the quality and integrity of our output. In a ventral vagal state where we can be ourselves, our endeavors become less strenuous, and our creations flow more abundantly.

---

* Polyvagal Insight 4: The Power of Social Connection and Co-Regulation

Chapter 12

From Surviving to Thriving with Parkinson's Disease

Case Overview

> **SSP PROVIDER:** Liz Charles, MD. Website: sensitiveapproach .co.uk
>
> **CLINICAL DISCIPLINE AND FOCUS:** Medical doctor with a deep neuroscience focus on understanding features related to trauma, chronic illness, and dysregulation of the ANS
>
> **OTHER THERAPEUTIC MODALITIES AND EXPERTISE:** Sensitive Approach: Client at the Core, PVT, Betsy Polatin's *Humanual* exercises,[1] and Frank Corrigan's Deep Brain Reorienting
>
> **CLIENT:** Frank (a pseudonym) is a middle-aged male who was diagnosed (via the DaTscan) with Parkinson's disease (PD) six years prior to his work with Liz. He also has a history of complex trauma.
>
> **FEATURES/SYMPTOMS:** Shaking (tremors), muscle stiffness (rigidity), slow and unsteady movement, digestive problems, depression, anxiety, poor sleep quality and low energy, reduced facial expressivity (a common symptom of PD, often called a "masked" or "flat" face), difficulty with speech, and lack of vocal prosody

AUTONOMIC TENDENCY: Frank's primary experience is the shutdown state of dorsal vagal, expressed as lethargy and other features of depression such as social withdrawal and a lack of energy and enthusiasm. He frequently finds himself trapped in the cyclic defense loop, oscillating between sympathetic and dorsal vagal states.

ASSESSMENTS: Parkinson's Disease Questionnaire (PDQ-39), Hospital Anxiety and Depression Scale (HADS), Brain-Body Center Sensory Scales (BBCSS)

Client Description

Frank had received a diagnosis of PD six years earlier. PD is a progressive neurological condition affecting dopamine levels in the brain and causing symptoms in the body like stiffness and tremors that get worse over time. Prior to his symptoms worsening, he had been a conscientious financial consultant and in a committed relationship with the mother of his young daughter. He loved long-distance running due to the satisfaction of sensing his body and feeling stronger than his pain. And along the way he achieved multiple personal bests.

By the time he met Liz, however, his PD symptoms had progressed, and activities of daily living were becoming increasingly difficult. His social behavior was affected by his expressed symptoms of PD. He suffered from a mask-like facial expression common among PD patients and lacked the ability to spontaneously express appropriate and reciprocal facial expressions. Subconsciously, through neuroception, a flat face is experienced by others as a "don't come near" signal. And yet, behind this facial mask of apparent disinterest, Frank was longing to authentically engage with those around him.

Frank was living alone, reclusive, depressed, and worried about his future. He felt he was running out of options.

Through his own trauma work, Frank had studied PVT. He recognized that some of his PD symptoms were related to an autonomic state in addition to PD. He understood that clinical psychiatric symptoms can be caused by being stuck in a cyclic defense loop—oscillating continuously between a sympathetic and dorsal vagal state. He wondered whether SSP could help him and actively searched until he found Liz. During their first meeting he described SSP as his "last hope."

During their initial sessions, Frank recounted his experience of developmental trauma. He was unable to recall many memories before the age of 14, and the little he remembered was negative. He had been diagnosed with absence seizures (brief, sudden lapses of consciousness) at age 10 and took medication for this until age 19. He had struggled with his mental health at various points in his adult life and had been treated with medication and psychotherapy both during inpatient and outpatient care in a psychiatric hospital. He does not remember ever experiencing a feeling of safety. He described himself as having two parts: one was a fighter wanting to be fine; the other was fearful, desperate, and questioning why he was alive.

SSP Delivery Method

SSP Core was delivered remotely in twice-weekly one-hour online sessions over the course of six months. Liz was present virtually with Frank for every SSP session and observed him closely. The listening was carefully titrated by both of them working together to track his responses to the filtered music of SSP. Due to his hypersensitivity, his individual listening segments were at times very short, sometimes lasting about one and a half minutes.

The SSP's acoustic cues were designed to generate feelings of safety and biobehavioral responses of calming. Liz immediately recognized, however, that for Frank those cues were triggering vulnerability and destabilizing his autonomic state. It was necessary to resolve the disruptive impact before listening to more of SSP. In response to each disruption, Liz and Frank used co-regulation and various somatic activities to allow his ANS to calm before resuming his listening. As a result of this approach, his total listening time per session was in the range of 3 to 12 minutes.

Liz employed her clinical and intuitive skills to co-regulate with Frank to allow his autonomic reactivity to settle. She used regulating exercises which, together with her personal interactions and co-regulation, could stabilize Frank's autonomic state and enable recovery. Her authentic co-regulating cues of safety and accessibility were felt by Frank, even remotely through a screen.

This method, which Liz named the Sensitive Approach: Client at the Core, is described as an individualized and co-regulatory process based on the client's sensitivities and is effective for many clients with complex trauma and chronic illness. It involves microtitration of SSP, meaning that the client listens to very short segments. To achieve this, Liz pays close attention to each client's responses to the music to observe when their disruptions first begin. By helping them listen to the whispers of their nervous system before they became shouts, she is able to expose her clients to the "just right" amount of listening. This gives them the opportunity to experience better outcomes.

For Frank, each session was different, and his progress was not linear. Initially, he periodically experienced sudden tightening in the front of his torso in response to SSP. He and Liz used this as a reliable signal of destabilization and the need to titrate the amount of listening. When Frank experienced this feeling, he paused the music, and Liz encouraged him to recognize this as SSP working. She then guided him to use the different regulation activities they had shared to release the tension and to also use other techniques he had learned from Somatic Experiencing and qigong.

Over time, as a product of this "neural exercise," Frank's muscle tightening became less frequent and when it occurred, his recovery became rapid. As Frank moved through the listening, however, he experienced some difficult emotions. His handling of them became more central to his process. Liz supported him and encouraged him to express and release them as they emerged.

Frank's recovery required a combination of SSP, increased awareness of his sensations and behaviors associated with his autonomic tendencies, familiarity and practice of regulating activities, and co-regulation. All of these together enabled him to achieve better body-brain integration and regulation. It was Frank's seeking nature and diligent research that allowed him to cultivate this effective holistic approach.

Liz and Frank maintained ongoing contact while he continued to listen to SSP. After his first round of SSP Core, he listened to SSP Balance for maintenance. He then had a second round of SSP Core before more SSP Balance. Eighteen months after starting the initial SSP Core, Frank listened to SSP Core for the third time. After that, he regularly listened to SSP Balance as well as SSP Connect as part of his self-care routine. He continued to find that they helped him to access a more balanced state and relieve his symptoms.

The natural progression of PD is a downward trajectory of physical and psychological symptoms. However, since starting with SSP, this was not Frank's experience. After each successive round of SSP Core, he felt more flexible in his movement, and his mood improved. Although he still had PD, was unable to work, and needed to persevere with his regular regime of speech therapy, physical therapy, qigong, and meditation to sustain his progress, he was now biking 10 miles on an exercise bike three to five times per week and enjoying a much-improved mood and quality of life. He was sure that SSP had facilitated this because he could tell he was no longer stuck in a cycle of mobilized and immobilized defensive states.

Summary of Provider's Observations about the Client's Response to SSP

Liz's work with Frank had a deep impact on her. At the time, there was scant clinical experience of using SSP for PD so the process was exploratory and experimental. Liz was immediately interested in working with Frank due to the profound impact PD had on him at such a young age combined with his enthusiasm to explore the impact of his trauma and PD on his ANS. Although his body was closed off, his mind and attitude were very much open. His courage, despite such physical and mental shutdown, helped build the trust and motivation needed for their powerful collaboration.

An unexpected early reward was the almost instant return of Frank's facial expressivity. Even during the first listening session, after only one and a half minutes of listening, they shared their total delight in noticing that Frank's face was coming alive and was distinctly different from his previous flat expression. He could smile! By the second session he was making jokes, which caused great pleasure as he couldn't remember the last time he had done so.

The return of his SES was a shared joy for Liz and Frank, especially as they observed how the benefits extended to his family and friends. His changes in facial expressivity opened the door for co-regulation, which became a catalyst and fundamental component of his upward spiral of connection and transformation.* The profound impact of this on his life, both in scope and intensity, would have been unimaginable before.

Frank's rigidity and movement also quickly improved. In the second session, he suddenly felt so flexible that he stood up to show Liz how he could move and how excited he was. This improved freedom of movement continued to expand. On their seventh session, he was uncharacteristically late, but for a joyful reason. He had been out with friends and had even ridden his bicycle there. His social life had made him late! They laughed and celebrated how much he had changed in such a short time.

Another dramatic response to SSP was the change in Frank's auditory acuity. This could be tracked by the volume he selected for listening to SSP Core, which he reduced from 25 to 10 during the first hour of listening and ultimately settled at 13 for the rest of the listening. This was an unexpected benefit for Frank because he had been sensitive to sounds his whole life, with certain sounds being alarmingly loud, and yet he experienced difficulty hearing voices amid the background noise.† This kind of improvement reflected the effect of SSP on the SES, which contributes to middle ear muscle regulation.

---

* Polyvagal Insight 5: Autonomic State Impacts Social Cues

† Polyvagal Insight 6: Autonomic State, Vocal Intonation, and Middle Ear Muscle Regulation Mutually Influence Each Other

Over this same period, Frank experienced many other beneficial changes. His speech became clearer and his voice more resonant and prosodic. He had better internal awareness and a clearer connection to how he felt in each of his autonomic states. His digestion improved, and he had less constipation, which is a common symptom of PD. His mood also improved along with greater freedom to express his emotions, and he was able to reduce and eventually discontinue his antidepressants.

Frank continued to use the regulating exercises that he explored and practiced with Liz in their sessions. These formed a core part of his daily routine for self-care and regulation. His capacity to attain a calm connected ventral state was greatly improved. His emotional and physical gains made through SSP were sustained, including better sleep, less depression and anxiety, better connections with the people in his life, and fluidity of movement. His responses were more appropriate to the circumstances, and he faced challenges with greater confidence and agency.[*]

Assessments

The PDQ-39 showed improvement in Frank's scores for daily functioning, emotional well-being, and social interactions, moving from "moderate" pre-SSP to "very mild" post-SSP. Similarly, his HADS scores for anxiety and depression shifted from "moderate" to "normal." All of these improvements still held true 18 months later. Additionally, Frank's self-reported sensory sensitivities in the auditory, visual, tactile, and digestion categories on the BBCSS showed considerable reductions in all areas post-SSP.

Summary of Client's Reflections on Their Response to SSP

Since Frank's initial use of SSP, his quality of life was much improved, and he saw himself on an upward trajectory. He continued to make progress by repeating the SSP Pathways and focusing on autonomic balance with regulating activities, exercise, qigong, and meditation. While

---

[*] Polyvagal Insight 8: The ANS Is at the Core of Our Physical and Mental Wellness

he wasn't cured from PD, he experienced a significant reduction of symptoms associated with it when he was in a state of safety—fewer active tremors, greater fluidity of movement, and a more buoyant mood.

Significantly, Frank had not needed to increase his levodopa medication dose since he started SSP. Levodopa replenishes dopamine levels and, over time, some patients require increasing doses to maintain symptom control due to the progressive nature of the disease and the gradual loss of dopamine-producing cells in the brain. Soon after starting SSP the first time, Frank began reducing his antidepressant dose and eventually no longer needed it. His mood was more stable, and he slept well without waking during the night. He felt optimistic, had lost 65 pounds, and had a healthy social life with good friends and a girlfriend. His speech therapist noted that his voice was more prosodic, and his friends noticed he smiled more and had better eye contact.

These positive features were dampened when he felt under pressure, but in contrast to before SSP, when he was in a state of almost permanent shutdown, he could help himself return to a state of balance and connection. This greater flexibility and improved control of his nervous system responses helped him stop feeling like a victim.[*]

Before Frank began his work with Liz and SSP, he was preoccupied with his future and worried about his inevitable decline. Afterward, he sometimes forgot that he had PD. During these moments, he felt he was living a relatively normal and happy life. He summarized his experience by saying, "Before SSP, I was surviving. Now I am living."

Case Analysis with Dr. Porges

This case illustrates both the extreme sensitivity of the client's nervous system and the powerful effects of SSP. The client's initial reaction to SSP can offer insights into their potential for destabilization as well as how beneficial SSP may be for them. Liz cultivated co-regulation and trust with Frank and encouraged curiosity rather than fear about his nervous system responses and autonomic states. In this way, Frank learned to

---

[*] Polyvagal Insight 7: The ANS Can Be Retuned to Prioritize Connection and Well-Being

tune in to his physical and interoceptive signals, which gave him valuable understanding about his shifts between different physiological states. Because of Liz's skill and experience, she was able to encourage Frank to recognize his state shifts and empower him to pause the listening as necessary. Extreme care was taken throughout each session to make sure Frank's system was settled and ready for the input of SSP.

PD patients may exhibit physical responses to SSP such as overt muscle tightening or subtle changes in their facial expression. Responses such as these are crucial to notice and respect as they are important clues for titration. According to PVT, autonomic symptoms associated with PD, such as reduced facial expression and vocal intonation, can often be secondary to or "piggybacked" onto the disease, reflecting the nervous system's defensive adaptations rather than the actual disease itself. The combination of careful microtitration by Liz along with Frank's astute self-awareness allowed for these protective adaptations to release, leading to significant reductions in his PD symptoms and a much-improved quality of life.

Co-Regulation, Predictability, and Agency

In this case study, co-regulation provided the foundation for Frank to experience the benefits of SSP. Co-regulation enabled his and Liz's nervous systems to spontaneously engage, resulting in the sense of trust that comes with predictability, agency, and a reciprocal relationship. Predictability came from the familiar pattern of their sessions and in the knowing that while dysregulation or muscle contraction might occur, it would also resolve. Agency existed in Frank knowing that his decisions about the listening and regulation activities would be respected. He had a voice in expressing both his negative and positive feelings. Along this journey, their relationship flourished with shared compassion, humor, respect, and joy.

Frank's process of change was an evolution. SSP and his work with Liz illustrates that social nourishment and support of and from others makes one more adaptable and flexible.* His clinical experiences with SSP and Liz formed an efficient and effective neural exercise. SSP acted as an accelerant in fostering co-regulation and connection between Frank's and Liz's nervous systems, and their mutual attunement supported the efficacy of SSP.

Release of Muscle Tension Related to PD

Rigidity and periodic involuntary muscle tightening are common symptoms of PD. This rigidity can affect many muscles, such as those of the face, causing the flat facial affect, or "mask," seen in PD patients. Periodic muscle tightening often affects the torso and limbs—experienced as tremors, spasms, rigidity, and problems with gait—and can be on one side of the body more than the other.

SSP encouraged a release from the cyclic defense loop and the emergence of the features of the SES. For instance, Frank's face dramatically came alive early in the listening, and his voice became more expressive. This indicates how his SES had been dormant due to the overwhelming autonomic threat of the disease but flourished when this diminished.

Additionally, his periodic muscle contractions became less frequent—they occurred half or a third less often—and when they did occur, they released much more quickly. As Frank's rigidity and tremors reduced, he also became more flexible, both physically and emotionally. The improvement in his facial expressivity and flexibility occurred when Frank was in a connected ventral state. Along with the episodic improvements directly related to the SSP listening, there was an accumulated improvement in his baseline levels of functioning in all aspects of his life.

Titration and Interoception

Titration of SSP is more art than science. The goal is to find the "just right" amount of listening to allow a positive response to emerge while avoiding destabilization. This can be helped by the improved interoception that seems to occur as SSP listening progresses. Interoception is the internal sense of our bodily sensations that are conveyed via sensory

---

* Polyvagal Insight 4: The Power of Social Connection and Co-Regulation

pathways, including the vagus nerve. Remember that roughly 80 to 90 percent of vagal fibers are sensory and provide information on the state of the viscera to the brain. It has been shown that an increase in vagal tone is correlated with interoceptive awareness.[2]

In polyvagal terms, interoception can also provide greater awareness of the changes associated with physiological states. Frank became more familiar and less fearful of the sensations related to state changes. He could then use this improved awareness to signal a need to pause the music and choose exercises to release any muscle tension and stabilize his body. Befriending his body this way and learning how it was reacting to the input of SSP taught him to be better attuned to his interoceptive signals. This strengthened autonomic feedback loops, enabling him to flexibly move in and out of states appropriately.*

Repeating SSP for Sustained Benefit for Symptoms of Chronic Disease

Perhaps due to his PD, Frank has continued to benefit from repeated SSP rounds since the ongoing disease process is a continuous trigger. This is different from complex trauma in which the nervous system continues to be impacted by hypersensitivities and hypervigilance, but the main assault on the nervous system occurred in the past.

Stimulating the Vagus Nerve via a Vagus Nerve Stimulator or SSP

PD patients may be prescribed a vagal nerve stimulator (VNS), which provides direct electrical stimulation to the vagus nerve. It can be considered a prosthesis because it augments the function of the vagus nerve. This can be helpful in the moment for reducing symptoms, but it may not create long-term change. In general, when the VNS is turned off, so are the positive responses.

In contrast, the experience of SSP is a neural exercise. It trains and increases the capacity to return to an engaged, ventral vagal state more easily, and the ANS is incrementally optimized. Even after SSP

---

* Polyvagal Insight 2: Autonomic States Bias Our Feelings, Thoughts, and Behaviors

is complete, when one is engaging naturally in the world, the upward spiral of a connected state begetting a connected state is strengthened.

Giving and receiving cues of safety, being aware of one's state, and regularly using regulating tools and activities to regain balance are ways to support and extend the neural exercise of strengthening vagal tone. This increases resilience to stress, makes it easier to recover from triggers, and provides better access to social engagement. These all optimize the experience of being a human and can lead to a better quality of life—as they did for Frank. This is just what was hoped for in the development of SSP—that when the portal of the SES was opened, it would remain open and flourish via the reinforcement of social stimulation.

Implications for Daily Life

Chronic illness is a common and stressful experience that significantly impacts the individual and their loved ones. Unfortunately, a secondary suffering often emerges in the form of a downregulated SES triggered by the illness. However, PVT can provide hope to patients and their caregivers by offering approaches to mitigate these additional symptoms that become attached to chronic illness. The approaches include connection, co-regulation, regulation practices to achieve a state of calmness and safety, and learning to understand and appreciate the protective functions of one's own nervous system. These are small steps, but they can make a big difference in one's relationship with their illness and ultimately improve one's quality of life.

Chapter 13

Navigating Gender Identity and Selective Mutism

Case Overview

SSP PROVIDER: Kelly Melhorn, MA, BCaBA, founder and owner of Selective Mutism H.E.L.P. Website: smhelp.org

CLINICAL DISCIPLINE: Kelly specializes in assisting children and teenagers with selective mutism (SM), which she became passionate about after her own daughter was diagnosed with SM at age 4 ½. SM is an anxiety disorder marked by a consistent inability to speak in certain social situations where speaking is expected, such as at school, even though the person can speak in other settings, like at home. It is not a matter of choice or refusal; rather, the person genuinely cannot speak in these triggering environments due to fear and panic.

OTHER THERAPEUTIC MODALITIES AND EXPERTISE: Behavioral analytic interventions, polyvagal-informed approach

CLIENT: Kai is a 14-year-old boy who lives in a small Midwestern town in the US with his parents, both naturalized US citizens originally from Vietnam. His mother arrived as a refugee in 1994, while his father came in 2007. English is the primary language spoken at home, although Kai also grew up speaking Vietnamese. Kai began seeing Kelly when he was 12 years old. At the time, he was using his birth name and identified with the pronouns she/they. He was navigating questions about his gender identity and coping with SM.

FEATURES/SYMPTOMS: SM, gender dysphoria, anxiety, depression, self-harm, and suicidal ideation. Gender dysphoria is a profound and persistent discomfort arising from a mismatch between a person's assigned gender at birth and their true, self-identified gender. Transgender and nonbinary persons may experience significant gender dysphoria, often from an early age, leading to feelings of confusion, shame, anxiety, and challenges in social interactions.

AUTONOMIC TENDENCY: The cyclic defense loop, an oscillation between sympathetic and dorsal vagal states

ASSESSMENTS: Patient Health Questionnaire-9 (PHQ-9)

Client Description

Kai was a precocious learner who excelled in reading and math and was typically a year or two ahead of his peers. It came as a surprise to his parents when he began experiencing intense anxiety about speaking in front of his class in fifth grade, at age 10. Kelly learned from Kai's mother that he was a shy person and had experienced a delay in expressive language development for which he underwent speech therapy from ages 2 to 5. He also saw an occupational therapist (OT) when he was 5 to address retained primitive reflexes.

Kai was extremely shy with certain people, but this experience in fifth grade was different. Signs of social anxiety became more evident during that school year. In situations where speech was expected, Kai would freeze, become mute, avoid eye contact, and sometimes cry. He seemed to devote all his energy to avoiding social situations. To address his challenges, his mother initiated the process to implement an individualized education plan (IEP) at school, including services to enhance emotional regulation and social language skills. Looking back, his parents believe that Kai began struggling with his gender identity around the same time that he began avoiding social situations.

By seventh grade, when he was 12, Kai was grappling with academic pressure, parental conflicts, and emotional distress as he navigated the disconnect between his assigned gender as a female and his true gender identity as a male. A falling out with his best friend over his gender identity exacerbated his distress, leading to a reluctance and eventual inability to speak in certain situations.

In January, his anxiety intensified, and Kai became more withdrawn from his parents. They discovered that he was experiencing self-harm and suicidal ideation. In response, his mother began seeking additional support for him.

Kai's mother found Kelly on Facebook and contacted her about Kai's SM. Kelly started working with Kai in February of his seventh-grade school year. By then, he had become more selective about those he felt comfortable speaking around. Apart from his family, there were only two or three teachers and four to six kids at school whom he trusted. He also experienced significant levels of anger, though he couldn't pinpoint its origin, and occasional constipation.

Kelly and Kai agreed to meet weekly for 30-minute virtual sessions. Kelly took the time to get to know Kai. She aimed to be someone who Kai could trust and connect with, and then help him discover his priorities and develop resilience, positive thinking, and coping strategies. Initially, Kai chose to have his camera on, but his microphone off, communicating only by nodding. Due to his anxiety, he was unable to answer a forced-choice question, respond by writing in the chat box, or indicate choices with his fingers.

The following month, Kai informed his family that he no longer wished to use his feminine given name. He requested to be called Kai and to use the pronouns he/him.

His parents supported his decision, but Kai continued to engage in self-harm. Concerned, they reached out to a local psychiatric facility where he underwent a psychological evaluation using the Behavior Assessment System for Children-3 (BASC-3). The results revealed difficulties in adaptability, social skills, and functional communication along with high levels of withdrawal. It was recommended that Kai participate in a four-week outpatient program for anxiety at the local hospital during which Kelly continued to provide weekly support. Although Kai learned to recognize his anxiety triggers and developed some coping skills, his interactions with the medical staff were difficult. They described him as stoic, disengaged, and resistant to typical conversation and age-appropriate social interactions.

Three months later, in July, with Kelly's consistent support, Kai began to respond with one- or two-word answers to direct questions from peers, his family, and Kelly. Gradually, he started initiating conversations with her, often with playful comments and observations. It became evident that Kai thrived when he felt a sense of connection, validation, and the freedom to communicate at his own pace.* Kelly also observed that his sense of humor emerged in relaxed and low-pressure situations. She recommended that his parents encourage his interests, provide positive feedback, and avoid pressuring him to speak.

Following Kelly's advice, Kai's parents granted him more autonomy over his daily routine and activities. Initially, he became more engaged in socializing through apps on his phone. He then began attending group meetings with peers who were also navigating being transgender. This involvement boosted Kai's confidence, gave him a sense of being understood, and improved communication between him and his parents.

However, after months without self-harm, Kai had another episode two weeks into eighth grade, at age 13. His mother responded with empathy and care, and Kai revealed that this cutting incident was triggered by rejection from school peers and academic pressure from his father.

Although this self-harm incident was distressing, the resulting understanding and support Kai received from his mom and Kelly helped him stop self-harming and led to significant improvements. He became more verbal with Kelly and his speech therapist at school, whom he saw weekly as part of his IEP. Kai also became actively involved at school and in the community, joining a theater program, participating in social gatherings

---

* Polyvagal Insight 4: The Power of Social Connection and Co-Regulation

with peers, and improving his verbal communication. Additionally, he started helping elementary students with math for his mom's tutoring company. Academically, with his parents easing off the pressure to achieve straight As and Bs, Kai mostly did well.

SSP Delivery Method

In December of Kai's eighth-grade year, at age 13, 10 months after they began working together, he started SSP with Kelly. She had been talking to him and his parents about PVT, his own autonomic tendencies, and how SSP could help retune his nervous system toward a more connected ventral state. Having built a trusting relationship with Kelly, Kai and his parents were excited to try this new therapy. Given Kai's history of anxiety, self-harm, and suicidal ideation, Kelly proceeded with caution (similar to what was described in chapter 8).

Kai listened to 10 minutes of SSP Core during his weekly sessions with Kelly. He chose to have his camera and microphone turned off, while Kelly kept her camera on so he could feel connected to her. He also listened for 10 minutes during his weekly in-person appointment with his OT, who worked with him on retained primitive reflexes and auditory sensitivities that Kelly had noticed.

Kelly selected 10 minutes as the initial listening duration due to Kai's history of anxiety and self-harm. She watched carefully for any signs of dysregulation, which would have indicated a need to pause, but Kai responded well to the 10-minute listening sessions, showing no signs of dysregulation. He reported feeling less tension and noticed that his breathing was deeper both during and after the listening.

Despite his initial reluctance to involve his parents in the SSP process, after four months, Kai wanted his mom present while he listened. They engaged in bouncing balls back and forth, which helped foster a sense of connection and support during the therapy. With his mom now included, Kai listened three to five days a week for 10 minutes each session, completing the full SSP Core program in April.

Summary of Provider's Observations about the Client's Response to SSP

In addition to the progress Kai had made through the polyvagal approach before starting SSP—such as speaking in class, joining a Genders and Sexualities Alliances (GSA) group, and participating in community theater—he became noticeably more independent and comfortable speaking with people both during and after SSP. During his sessions with Kelly, Kai showed increased focus, confidence, and verbal engagement. His voice grew stronger, he responded more effectively to open-ended questions, and his answers became more detailed. Kai's auditory hypersensitivities decreased, and he no longer complained about ambient noises that had previously distracted him.*

After the first hour of listening, Kai felt comfortable enough to ask his mother for help with his science homework, something he had previously found challenging. By the end of Hour 2 of SSP, he performed in his first theater role and delivered five lines. Later, he successfully auditioned for a part in the school play and joined a weekly community improv class.

By Hour 4 of SSP, Kai began to show increased flexibility, openness, and willingness to step out of his comfort zone, especially in social settings. He agreed to be randomly assigned to peer groups in class—a notable change from his previous preference for being matched with specific classmates. During a virtual research class, he consistently kept his camera on and engaged actively in the class chat. Kai found himself enjoying his grammar class more and more. To his mother's surprise, he began to prefer group class participation over one-on-one sessions with the teacher. At his church group, he joined in games and responded to questions with ease—behaviors he would have struggled with before.

Kai was also open to the idea of switching schools for high school in ninth grade rather than remaining at his current school. This meant attending open houses at prospective schools and successfully completing

---

* Polyvagal Insight 6: Autonomic State, Vocal Intonation, and Middle Ear Muscle Regulation Mutually Influence Each Other

an in-person interview. He began demonstrating more independence, including biking to local stores, taking public transportation, and meeting friends outside his home.* During a two-week theater camp, he made a new friend and even proactively showed Kelly a picture of the two of them together.

After completing SSP, Kai started smiling and maintaining better eye contact.† He began using his voice more frequently and grew increasingly comfortable speaking and singing. Two months after completing SSP, Kelly and Kai engaged in a continuous 19-minute conversation—an impressive improvement from his previous sessions, where he had only spoken a few words or sentences. Additionally, he planned his own birthday party and invited three friends to attend.

In late August, at age 14, Kai started his ninth-grade year at his new school and attended several welcome events where he actively engaged in open-ended questions—something that used to be challenging for him. During the first week, he confidently introduced himself, shared fun facts, and asked questions of his new classmates. His physics teacher observed his active participation during a lab investigation, and a math teacher was so impressed with Kai that he invited him to join his higher-level class. Since completing SSP and switching schools, Kai's motivation for math homework, note-taking, and textbook highlighting has significantly improved. Additionally, his friendship with his friend from theater camp grew, and they attended a second theater camp together.

After SSP, Kai's overall anxiety and depression lessened. He formed more genuine connections with others, and his relationship with his parents improved. He also became more at ease with his transgender identity and felt more comfortable expressing himself authentically.

Assessments

Although Kelly had already been working intensively with Kai, she administered the PHQ-9 before and after SSP. The PHQ-9 screens for

---

* Polyvagal Insight 2: Autonomic States Bias Our Feelings, Thoughts, and Behaviors

† Polyvagal Insight 5: Autonomic State Impacts Social Cues

and assesses the severity of depression symptoms, with scores ranging from 0 to 27, where higher scores indicate greater severity of depression. Kai's pre-SSP score was 8 and his post-SSP score was 5. Both scores fell within the 5–9 range, indicating "mild depressive disorder." A score of 4 or less would indicate the absence of depressive disorder.

Summary of Client's and Parents' Reflections on Client's Response to SSP

Kai reported experiencing less anxiety and feeling more at ease during social interactions since completing SSP.[*] This improvement was evident in his successful start to high school, his positive theater experiences, and his active participation in improv class. He also described his relationship with his parents as being smoother.

Kai's ability to focus his attention improved, enabling him to join and succeed in an advanced math class and to remember his lines for theater productions. His mother noted, "At home, Kai seems more relaxed, less stressed out about school work, and more open in his communication." Although challenges with emotional regulation persisted, she observed a positive change in his confidence. Kai began openly communicating with his father whenever he needed a break from homework or no longer needed his father's assistance. This significant shift in their dynamic led to a more enjoyable home life for everyone.

Kai's family supported him as a transgender male. His mother educated herself on gender identity and attended several parent coaching sessions. At school, Kai felt supported through his participation in a GSA group, which helped him express his true self more easily with friends and family. His mother asked if he would like to start hormone blockers but, so far, Kai has chosen to decline this option. She observed that Kai was using more masculine body language, speaking in a slightly lower voice, and sporting a shorter hairstyle.

Thanks to acceptance, co-regulation, various therapies, and SSP, Kai's nervous system became more regulated and open to connecting with

---

[*] Polyvagal Insight 1: Autonomic State Functions as an Intervening Variable

himself and others. This progress enabled him to pursue his passions and led to a more fulfilling, authentic, and enriched life.*

Case Analysis with Dr. Porges

Through the lens of PVT, SM is a manifestation of a destabilized ANS. In defensive states, access to the SES is limited, reducing speech and spontaneous engagement. Triggers for SM vary by person, but common factors include anxiety, trauma, family stress, situational factors like moving house or changing schools, and speech and language difficulties. PVT suggests that all of these factors share a common impact on the ANS.

Symptoms associated with SM include an inability to speak in certain situations, retained primitive reflexes, auditory hypersensitivity, slow movements or speech, delayed reaction time, rigid or low muscle tone, digestive disorders, social anxiety, and poor interoception. These features may be linked to a "sluggish vagal brake"[1] causing delays in the activation or deactivation of different states including a ventral vagal state.

Poor regulation of the vagal brake can lead to difficulties in regulating autonomic states, impacting emotional regulation, social interactions, and overall nervous system functioning. This neurophysiological explanation sheds light on why individuals with SM may struggle to adapt to new social situations and experience periodic difficulties accessing neural control of the larynx and pharynx, essential for speech. A sluggish vagal brake also hinders innervation of the cranial nerves associated with SES, affecting facial expressivity, eye contact, prosody of voice, and the ability to process the sounds of human voice. This perspective clarifies that for people with SM, not speaking in certain situations is not a choice but is physiologically restricted due to the state of their ANS.

As with any multifaceted condition, individuals with SM exhibit unique combinations of symptoms that vary over time, mirroring shifts in autonomic states. When the metabolic demands of defensive states exceed the body's and nervous system's capacity, symptoms may peak.

---

* Polyvagal Insight 7: The ANS Can Be Retuned to Prioritize Connection and Well-Being

Kai's symptom constellation included retained primitive reflexes, auditory hypersensitivity, anxiety, and occasional constipation. These were all signs that his ANS was downregulated, and his nervous system was in a state of chronic defensiveness. Being in a defensive survival state also hinders access to higher cognition.

Gender Identity and Safety

Kai described how his gender identity journey evolved over time, moving from "comfort with being a girl, to some discomfort, to embracing a nonbinary identity, to leaning toward the gender identity of male, and ultimately identifying as a trans male" by the end of seventh grade. He currently feels more at ease with his gender than ever before.

The path to finding comfort within one's mind and body for those whose gender does not align with the one they were assigned at birth can be confusing and difficult. But Kai seems to be navigating it well. Feeling at ease with his gender and receiving love and support from the people in his life will provide greater autonomic capacity and flexibility. This will allow him to regulate his emotions effectively, enhance his social interactions, and fully express his inherent brilliance.

The outside world is filled with cues of threat, particularly in environments like school and family, where signals of evaluation abound. One's inner world, too, can signal threat when one's true identity is at odds with the gender one is assigned at birth as can be the case in gender dysphoria.

Individuals with gender dysphoria can experience a broad spectrum of emotions and behaviors ranging from feelings of confusion, anxiety, and distress to moments of self-discovery, empowerment, and relief. When distressful, gender dysphoria can lead to a cyclic defense loop, where one oscillates between an activated sympathetic state and a withdrawn dorsal state, creating a vortex of emotional and physiological dysregulation.

When one is trapped in this cycle, it's difficult to escape it and be able to feel safe or to be authentically connected to others and with the joys of life. But coping with distress from external and internal sources is achievable when there are "islands of safety"—moments of feeling at ease with and acceptance from others, allowing our bodies to find calm. For Kai, his secure havens were his friends, family, Kelly, and theater.

Passions Align with Purpose

Passions often reflect what one's nervous system needs and appreciates. Kai's passion was theater, and it provided many opportunities to deepen self-awareness and hone his social engagement skills.

The experience of acting is a complex neural exercise of the SES. In the realm of psychotherapy, theater and psychodrama are outlets for expressing and exploring emotions. By delving into specific feelings to convey them to the audience, actors develop a heightened sense of interoception—the ability to perceive and interpret bodily signals from internal organs and respond appropriately. This skill, integral to the brain-body connection, contributes to one's sense of embodiment and self-understanding.

Many actors, including those who grapple with social anxiety, find comfort on the stage due to its predictable structure. Kai found this to be true and valued the social engagement and co-regulation within the community.

The Immigrant Experience and Polyvagal Parenting

Immigrant parents, facing uncertainty in a new country, often push their children to succeed, viewing education as the key to a better life. This can place a heavy burden on kids, and when the pressure becomes excessive, it can actually hinder their ability to learn.

Kai was a good student and very smart, but he would go into a dorsal shutdown state when the pressure was too great. He would procrastinate and had difficulties with his schoolwork. This makes sense from a polyvagal perspective. Chronic defensiveness compromises brain functions vital for learning.

A turning point for Kai was when his parents reduced their pressure on him for academic performance, focused instead on his interests and strengths, and gave him more independence. Quickly, Kai's concentration and motivation improved, he was able to do better in school, and he was invited to join higher-level classes. He now communicates more freely, feels more authentically himself, and is able to be more present in his relationships with his family.

His parents continue to confront ingrained expectations, but when they observed Kai struggling, they prioritized his happiness, prompting them to adjust their approach. Though it's a learning process, they have adapted their parenting style to better support his needs. They now actively support his gender identity and emotional well-being, fostering rapport and connection, and responding sensitively to the cues of his nervous system.

Implications for Daily Life

Threats to the nervous system can take various forms. External experiences such as abuse or neglect, war, or medical procedures are commonly acknowledged as traumas. However, internal experiences, while not as explicit and often unseen, can also be potent signals of threat to the nervous system. In addition to more recognized examples like disease, pain, and fatigue, there are also less obvious ones such as hormonal fluctuations, cognitive impairments, and gender dysphoria, among others. It's important to notice and recognize the profound impact that triggers from the internal landscape can have on the nervous system. Regardless of the origin of the distress and dysregulation, using regulation strategies (like SSP and those outlined in chapter 4) can help alleviate suffering and generate hope.

Chapter 14

Unexpected SSP Response Alters the Clinical Arc of Recovery

Case Overview

SSP PROVIDER: Deirdre Stewart, LPC, SEP, BCN, vice president of Trauma Resolution Services for Meadows Behavioral Healthcare. Website: themeadows.com

CLINICAL DISCIPLINE: Mental health counselor, educator, and trainer supporting healing from complex trauma and addiction

OTHER THERAPEUTIC MODALITIES AND EXPERTISE: Neurofeedback, NeuroAffective Relational Model, Somatic Experiencing, and somatic and attachment-focused EMDR

CLIENT: Marie (a pseudonym) is a 36-year-old married female who has been in recovery for drug and alcohol addiction for more than 10 years with intensive support from the Meadows on an outpatient basis. The Meadows is an established and highly respected facility that offers many therapeutic modalities that are integrated to support people in overcoming addiction, heal unresolved emotional trauma, and develop the tools they need to transform their lives.

FEATURES/SYMPTOMS: Marie has a significant history of trauma, including birth, shock, and developmental trauma.

She suffers from addiction, migraines, mood instability, and panic attacks. She has been diagnosed with bipolar II and has experienced long-term stabilization from medication, which she continues to take.

AUTONOMIC TENDENCY: Marie often fluctuated between the sympathetic and dorsal vagal states of the cyclic defense loop. At times of more sympathetic dominance, she experienced perseveration, anxiety, overwhelm, and panic attacks. At times of more dorsal influence, blunted affect, flat facial expressivity, depression, shame, and numbing. When arousal and attention were within her window of tolerance, she could experience a blended state of sympathetic and ventral vagal states.

ASSESSMENTS: Pre- and post-SSP Quantitative Electroencephalography (qEEG) testing

Client Description

Marie was born in a small, remote town in Washington to a 16-year-old who unexpectedly became pregnant and decided to put Marie up for adoption. Marie was adopted at three days old and knows very little about her biological parents. Her brother, two years younger, was also adopted, and both were raised with strong conservative religious beliefs.

Described by Marie as "narcissistic," her adoptive father was neglectful, verbally and emotionally abusive, critical, and demanding. Additionally, he was unchecked in his sexual energy. Marie wonders if she might have been exposed to sexual abuse during her preverbal years. While she has no explicit memories, her somatic memories and panic attacks suggest that something may have happened.

Marie's adoptive mother was nurturing and supportive, but she tended to lean on Marie for emotional support as she experienced distress in her marriage due to her husband's extramarital affairs.

Now a 36-year-old woman, Marie actively engages in therapies to continue her recovery from trauma and its effects, including addiction. She struggled with drug and alcohol addiction from ages 14 to 26 and has been in remission for over 10 years. Additionally, she is recovering from disordered eating behavior. As a child, from ages 4 to 8, Marie experienced pica, a condition characterized by a craving to eat nonfood substances like plaster, paper, or clay. She also struggled with narcolepsy, which once prevented her from retaining employment and maintaining daily functioning. After undergoing 25 sessions of neurofeedback training, she was able to successfully manage this condition and has been employed in her current role for over seven years.

Marie attends weekly therapy sessions to address interpersonal disturbances, a negative self-concept, and regulation challenges and to continue building resilience. She has a diagnosis of bipolar II, marked by hyperexcitability and hypersensitivities and experiences dissociation, migraines, and panic attacks.

Despite facing extensive adversity, Marie is exceptionally bright and possesses considerable internal resources. Her ability to stay present and flexibly shift states helps her manage day-to-day challenges effectively and, overall, she feels relatively content in her current life. Marie hoped that SSP would further her healing and growth as she wanted to overcome her moderate-to-severe sugar addiction, decrease her hypersensitivities, and shift the way she relates to herself and others. Her goals were to experience greater peace, less reactivity, and more self-love and compassion.

SSP Delivery Method

Deirdre had supported Marie with various therapeutic modalities at the Meadows for over 10 years. During this time they developed a close and trusting relationship based on consistent and compassionate care. Marie was well-acquainted with the Meadow's comprehensive support network, including access to other skilled therapists and a range of facilities. This familiarity and access gave her confidence in her ongoing healing journey. For Deirdre, knowing that Marie had these robust support options also provided a sense of reassurance.

This was Marie's third time undergoing SSP with Deirdre. The first experience, at the beginning of 2019, led to increased vitality and what Marie described as a "clean windshield effect"—the world appeared brighter.

The second SSP experience, which took place in March of 2023, resulted in lasting improvements including enhanced embodiment, a greater ability to connect with others, and a reduction in social anxiety, self-doubt, and overarousal.

SSP Core was delivered using the SEGAN approach developed by Ana do Valle, just as it had been the previous two times. At the Meadows, this method of SSP delivery complements their extensive range of therapeutic modalities. SEGAN involves daily 90-minute individual sessions over five consecutive days, each including one hour of listening to SSP Core. Deirdre was always present to support Marie, helping her track sensations, affect, and impulses while using images to create meaning. Marie chose to paint with watercolors during the listening sessions with Deirdre.[1]

Each listening session went smoothly, and Marie appeared calm and settled throughout. However, between her daily sessions, she experienced intense sympathetic activation, a reaction that had not occurred during her previous SSP experiences. On the evenings following Hours 3 and 4, she described feeling both overstimulated and exhausted, alternating between yelling and being on the verge of tears, sometimes experiencing both emotions simultaneously. As the week progressed, her mood became increasingly unstable, and she felt more agitated. During these distressing times, Marie was grateful for the support of her husband and the easy access to Deirdre, who provided support and reassurance over the phone.

Summary of Provider's Observations about the Client's Response to SSP

Marie experienced significant distress and discomfort during and after the week of her SSP sessions, and she required ongoing reassurance and support from her long-term therapist. Despite these challenges, Marie navigated through them and ultimately saw a positive outcome. Her executive functioning along with her complex cognitive processing and working memory improved. Her orienting response gradually shifted from defensive to more exploratory, a change that had been evolving since her first round of SSP. Additionally, her facial expressions have softened and become more expressive, her eye contact has improved, and her overall affect appears brighter and more animated. She has more energy and is generally more upregulated.

However, this third round of SSP activated Marie's nervous system more intensely than the previous two and created some ongoing challenges. Her primary coping strategy—dissociation or "checking out"—was significantly reduced. Without this long-standing coping mechanism that she has relied on, she experienced more "intense emotions" and felt less able to cope. With skilled therapeutic support to address these heightened feelings of anger and increased sadness, Marie navigated these emotional challenges to ultimately achieve positive change. This ongoing reorganization in Marie's brain was measured by qEEG.

This case highlighted two key learnings about SSP delivery. First, it emphasized the importance of starting SSP early in a client's addiction treatment program, which typically involves a one-month inpatient stay. Starting earlier would allow more time for full integration and processing of the experience. Although Marie's shifts were ultimately positive, they required adjustments in strategy and additional support. A more gradual, titrated approach to SSP might have helped mitigate the destabilizing effects and facilitated a smoother integration of her new way of being in the world.

Another key learning is that SSP is not a one-time intervention for everyone. Each round of SSP can bring a deepening and shifting of both the client's physiology and their brain's organization. Marie's reduced ability to buffer against incoming stimuli will, over time, enable her to be more present and regulated and move away from a freeze state. In the interim, she will continue to benefit from Deirdre's therapeutic support and attuned presence.

Marie is continuing her journey of recovery and healing. While the third round of SSP was challenging, it prompted her to explore new ways of engaging socially. Given her shifts in auditory processing and heightened arousal, ongoing support and integration will be beneficial for Marie. The plan includes the possibility of administering SSP for a fourth time in a few months to further support her progress.

Assessments

Pre- and post-SSP qEEGs were conducted to assess the effects of SSP on Marie's brain wave activity. Observable changes were documented in the four pre- and post-SSP qEEG measurements. Penijean Gracefire, LMHC, BCN, qEEG-D, a neural frequency analyst specializing in 3D brain imaging technology and a consultant for the Meadows's neurofeedback team, conducted and reviewed Marie's qEEG analysis.

The pre- and post–SSP "eyes closed" frequency distribution, a measure of how the brain allocates resources, provides insight into habitual activation patterns. In Marie's pre-SSP map, the highest activity was observed in delta waves. Delta waves are associated with cortical deafferentation during mental tasks, which suggests inhibition of sensory inputs to enhance internal concentration.[2] For Marie, the persistent surplus of delta waves may have functioned as a stress management strategy, helping her to mitigate social and sensory demands from her external environment while processing emotional and cognitive tasks.

In Marie's post-SSP analysis, there was a significant decrease in delta activity and a noticeable increase in beta and gamma frequencies. These findings would indicate that Marie's brain is spending less time in slower frequencies and more time in faster frequencies, resulting in upregulation, enhanced processing speed, and productivity.[3]

Clinically, the excess delta observed pre-SSP allowed Marie to buffer incoming demands and auditory stimuli. Based on her history and self-report, this likely reflects a long-standing dissociative strategy similar to the dorsal vagal response described within Polyvagal Theory. SSP appears to have reorganized her brain's functioning, reducing this buffering effect. As a result, Marie now engages more actively in the present moment and interacts more fully with her environment, marking a significant shift in her brain's coping strategy.

The pre- and post-SSP "eyes open" images and Z-score analysis of frequency distribution reveal a shift in activation. Marie initially showed higher engagement in the rear left auditory cortex, which shifted to higher engagement on the right side post-SSP. This indicates a reorganization and reprioritization of her brain functioning.

Marie's pre- and post-SSP "eyes closed" alpha peak frequency scores indicate a more balanced auditory functioning post-SSP, although a slightly slower processing speed was observed. Her left frontal alpha frequency decreased, suggesting reduced avoidance and increased engagement. While this change is positive, the heightened sensory input presented is challenging.[4]

Finally, the pre- and post-SSP "eyes open" alpha peak frequency scores demonstrate that Marie's brain is less compartmentalized and exhibits more network synchrony. These findings are associated with improved cortical integration and are also linked to enhanced emotional processing of social cues.[5]

Marie's reported feelings of overwhelm during and after SSP primarily stemmed from changes in her ability to regulate incoming stimuli. With reduced right frontal avoidance mechanisms and diminished gating capacity, she became more sensitive to all inputs. This shift had two significant effects: she was less able to dissociate from experiences, sensations, or emotions, leading to heightened sensory experiences, and she spent more time in higher frequencies (beta and gamma), resulting in increased hypervigilance in the back-parietal region, particularly in response to incoming sensory information.[6]

Summary of Client's Reflections on Their Response to SSP

Marie found this third round of SSP "much more challenging" than the previous two. Although she experienced the daily 90-minute sessions as resourcing and enjoyed her time with Deirdre and painting, she was surprised by the wider range of emotions that emerged between sessions and after completion. Processing and integrating these changes and emotions required significant time and effort. While the shifts ultimately proved positive, the initial destabilization was distressing and required unexpected additional support.

Marie experienced symptoms of destabilization, including nervous system activation, emotional volatility, such as bouts of crying and yelling, and agitation. She also struggled with losing her ability to dissociate, making it difficult to adjust to the changes in her internal experience. As she continues her journey, Marie is exploring new ways to navigate social interactions more effectively.

Despite these challenges, Marie was pleased to notice many positive changes. She was able to be more present in the here and now, and she was grateful to have successfully reduced her sugar cravings and consumption.* Her processing speed and clarity of thought improved, along with her sense of spatial orientation, which was a surprise. Her husband observed a significant improvement in her sense of direction and navigational abilities.

Other notable benefits to Marie from this round of SSP include freedom from panic attacks and a considerable reduction in her hypersensitivities. Her relationship with herself feels more grounded, and she navigates her relationships with others more positively by better connecting with her emotions and sensations. Marie can now connect with others without merging with them. She has also experienced an increase in self-love and compassion, which has helped her establish healthier boundaries with work, family, and friends. Recently, Marie's increased social engagement led to a new, meaningful friendship, marking a significant step forward in her personal growth.†

Marie remains hopeful that the shifts will lead to long-term positive outcomes. For her, the benefits outweigh the difficulties, as evidenced by her interest in undergoing SSP for a fourth time. Her case highlights that while SSP's effect may not always align with specific intentions, it consistently works to repattern the nervous system toward greater balance and resilience.

---

* Polyvagal Insight 8: The ANS Is at the Core of Our Physical and Mental Wellness

† Polyvagal Insight 7: The ANS Can Be Retuned to Prioritize Connection and Well-Being

Case Analysis with Dr. Porges

One notable aspect of this case is our ability to link Marie's autonomic and behavioral responses to SSP with the corresponding changes in her brain waves detected through qEEG. Additionally, her experience demonstrates how multiple applications of SSP can bring about different features and capabilities.

Marie felt completely overwhelmed after her third and most recent SSP experience. She described how she previously relied on a protective form of light dissociation, which served as an effective survival strategy by creating a barrier between herself and the outside world. However, after this round of SSP, that protective barrier was stripped away. Without it, she struggled to stay regulated with the unexpected influx of stimuli, with every external input feeling like an unwelcome intrusion.

The changes in brain wave patterns observed in the qEEG mapping were consistent with Marie's subjective experience. As detailed in the earlier "Assessments" section, over the five-day span between the pre- and post-SSP qEEG mapping sessions, Marie exhibited a significant decrease in delta brain wave activity. These slow brain waves reflect less sensory and motor input to the brain. Their reduction correlates with her previous capacity to inhibit sensory input and highlights the challenges she faced post-SSP in managing greater incoming stimuli.

Another qEEG observation was that, before SSP, Marie's brain exhibited a significant imbalance, with her alpha brain waves being notably higher in the left, relative to the right hemisphere auditory processing areas. After SSP, alpha activity became more fully synchronized between the two hemispheres. Typically, achieving a more balanced level of alpha brain wave activity correlates with greater autonomic flexibility, but this significant shift will take time to be accommodated by Marie's system.

The shift toward the right hemisphere in alpha brain waves may also indicate three other potential changes. First, it's conceivable that Marie had a left ear advantage before undergoing this round of SSP, and that her right ear became more balanced post-SSP. A right ear advantage is preferred because auditory input to the right ear is typically routed to the left hemisphere, which, in most individuals, is more specialized in language and speech processing. This shift could potentially enhance her hearing acuity and auditory processing ability.[*] Although Marie's auditory processing was not tested, it's worth noting that a SCAN-3 test often reveals improvements in auditory acuity and processing following SSP.[7]

The second change observed in Marie was a significant improvement in her navigational skills, despite long-standing difficulties in this area. The increased balance between her right and left temporal lobes suggests enhanced activity in the right parietal lobe, which is crucial for spatial memory, visual-spatial information processing, and navigation tasks.

The third improvement for Marie involves social processing, which tends to be more associated with the right hemisphere. In conjunction with the loss of her previous capacity to buffer incoming stimuli, it appears that Marie shifted toward a more externally focused approach. Marie had been accustomed to experiencing extreme social anxiety and frequently avoided social situations. However, after SSP, she noticed herself becoming more open and authentic, and she was able to forge a new, genuine friendship, which both surprised and delighted her.[†]

Buffers Aren't Selective

Survival instincts within our body and nervous system can create barriers and buffers to keep us safe and able to function when we meet challenging situations.[‡] However, these buffers aren't selective. In filtering out environmental stressors, negative emotions, and overwhelming sensations, they also block cues of safety, reassurance, and connection. As a result, this can lead to a sense of disconnection and feeling unmoored, similar to a shutdown dorsal vagal state.

Marie vividly described the energy required to maintain a professional demeanor, comparing it to a duck gliding smoothly across the

---

[*] Polyvagal Insight 6: Autonomic State, Vocal Intonation, and Middle Ear Muscle Regulation Mutually Influence Each Other

[†] Polyvagal Insight 4: The Power of Social Connection and Co-Regulation

[‡] Polyvagal Insight 2: Autonomic States Bias Our Feelings, Thoughts, and Behaviors

water while paddling furiously beneath the surface. Creating barriers between one's internal and external worlds and masking true emotions is exhausting, often leading to disconnection from both others and from oneself.

Chronic Defensiveness as a Feature of Addiction

Individuals with a history of trauma are often detached from their body, leading to a disconnection between the body and brain. While this detachment may be adaptive in acute situations, it can result in bodily numbness and cause the brain to create a narrative without accurate input from the body. This loss of connection often results in a chronic defensive state where the individual is trapped in a relentless cycle between sympathetic and dorsal vagal states, while the ventral vagal circuit remains inaccessible.

Addiction often arises when the ANS is stuck in a defensive state, leading individuals to rely on addictive substances and behaviors to reduce the discomfort that comes with these states. While these strategies may temporarily numb feelings of distress and physical pain, they fail to provide access to the ventral vagal state where true regulation and homeostasis occur. From a polyvagal perspective, addiction is viewed as an attempt to alleviate underlying feelings of threat, with the individual's actions reflecting a desperate search for safety. However, trying to achieve safety through addictive behaviors ultimately falls short, as true safety and a sense of well-being are only found through connection and social engagement.[8]

Multiple SSP Boosters Can Be Helpful

After completing SSP once, many clients report enhanced autonomic flexibility, which is further supported by their increased self-awareness and engagement in regulating activities (as discussed in chapter 4). This newfound flexibility often results in a profound and lasting shift in their life trajectory.

Some clients, however, find further benefit from repeating SSP. This was first observed in children, where exposure to external stressors like viruses, accidents, or shocks after completing SSP could sometimes push the ANS back into a defensive state, leading to compromised co-regulation and difficulties in self-regulation. Administering an SSP booster, often just a few listening sessions, showed promising results and was demonstrated to reset the ANS into regulation again.

As understanding deepened within the provider community, it became evident that SSP boosters also benefited individuals with trauma histories, particularly those with developmental trauma characterized by an adaptive disconnection between the body and brain. Providers reported that repeating SSP with these clients led to new outcomes, such as increased self-exploration and openness to bodily sensations. Over time, these individuals became more familiar with and consistent in achieving a connected, ventral vagal state, fostering greater resilience.

Marie has faced challenges integrating the changes from her third round of SSP. However, shifts in her autonomic state, behaviors, and brain wave activity indicate that she is increasingly able to engage socially and regulate her nervous system without relying on sugar. This suggests the emergence of a new neuroception of safety, potentially allowing her to break free from the cyclic defense loop and gain better access to social engagement and homeostasis.

Implications for Daily Life

Addiction is not a choice; it's an adaptive survival response to dysregulation. Individuals may turn to addictive substances or behaviors to seek relief from the chaos of sympathetic activation or the numbness and despair of dorsal vagal shutdown. While this approach may offer short-term comfort, it doesn't address the root cause of the dysregulation and may even deepen the nervous system's entrapment in a cyclic defense loop.

PVT offers a compassionate and nonjudgmental view of behaviors for anyone, recognizing that our thoughts, emotions, and behaviors result from the state of our nervous system. When the nervous system is supported and connected, it provides the platform for relief and new possibilities.

Chapter 15

COVID Recovery and a Renewed Relationship with Self

Case Overview

SSP PROVIDER: Jill Hosey, MSW, RSW. Website: jillianhosey.com

CLINICAL DISCIPLINE AND FOCUS: Jill is a clinical social worker and trauma therapist providing therapy to children, youth, and adults who are struggling with experiences of trauma, PTSD, attachment and developmental trauma, and dissociative disorders. Jill is the lead author of the "Combined Delivery Guidelines for EMDR and SSP."

OTHER THERAPEUTIC MODALITIES AND EXPERTISE: Eye movement desensitization and reprocessing therapy (EMDR), Deep Brain Reorienting (DBR), trauma-focused cognitive behavioral therapy (CBT), Sensorimotor Psychotherapy, and PVT. Jill is also knowledgeable about neurofeedback and the Alexander Technique (AT), although she does not use them with her clients.

CLIENT: Jill's history included migraines, irritable bowel syndrome, and childhood relational trauma. In the fall of 2022, when she became suddenly bedridden due to acute COVID, she assumed the roles of both therapist and client, delivering SSP to herself starting on the ninth day of her illness. Additionally, she engaged in neurofeedback on three afternoons after listening to SSP.

FEATURES/SYMPTOMS: Jill experienced severe COVID symptoms including brain fog, working memory struggles, fatigue, severe dizziness, inability to focus or concentrate, tachycardia, and severe gastrointestinal upset. These symptoms triggered her history of childhood relational and attachment trauma, causing feelings of powerlessness and a need to hide. She also experienced anxiety and depression, as well as anger toward her body due to her loss of control over it, and its failure to recover quickly.

Due to her childhood experiences, Jill had developed a self-protective habit of maintaining distance from others and herself. Facing severe COVID illness revealed to her the drawbacks of this approach, underscoring her reluctance to ask for help, show vulnerability, and practice self-compassion.

AUTONOMIC TENDENCY: Will attempt sympathetic first and then shift to dorsal vagal.

ASSESSMENTS: No formal assessments were utilized.

Client Description

As a clinician and EMDR trainer, Jill is used to helping and teaching other people. When her extreme symptoms of COVID came on rapidly, rendering her unable to get out of bed, she realized she needed to apply her knowledge, skills, and tools to help herself.

She suffered a complete loss of smell and taste, severe fatigue, body pain (even her skin hurt), a sore throat, chest pain and cough, severe headache, and stabbing eye pain. Of particular concern was her chest pain; her resting heart rate, already high at 100–120 bpm, now raced even faster with an irregular beat. By the third day of symptoms, she attempted to read a book but couldn't manage a full page, struggling to recall even the little she had read. This was markedly different from her usual response to illness.

By the ninth day, her symptoms shifted. Some of the original symptoms eased as new ones materialized. She had extreme dizziness. The ground underneath her seemed to be moving, and she had no balance. A heavy brain fog descended and with it came disorientation, an inability to concentrate, and problems with word recall and working memory. Worried, she tested herself by trying to read some chapters of a book on a therapeutic model she often taught. She couldn't remember any of it. She panicked—what if she didn't recover? She felt hopeless and fearful about what was to come.* Her felt sense of "me-ness" was challenged. How would she function? How could she work? Who even was she? She questioned the value of how she had constructed her sense of self in the world.

At this point, her fast heart rate and heart palpitations worsened, and she began experiencing sudden nausea and diarrhea. She wondered if she was experiencing vagus nerve dysfunction as that could explain her dizziness, and her heart, chest, and stomach difficulties. The little reading on COVID she could manage suggested she might be moving out of the acute phase and toward something more chronic like the Long COVID she was reading about.[1] The research mentioned vagus nerve stimulation as a potential treatment targeting inflammatory and immunological processes.[2] Jill immediately thought of SSP, which is patented as an acoustic vagus nerve stimulator and provides neural exercises to improve access to ANS balance and flexibility.

SSP Delivery Method

Despite the recommendation against self-delivery of SSP, Jill's symptoms, particularly her extreme dizziness, were so worrisome she believed she needed to act quickly. She had previously listened to SSP Core twice— first in short increments and later in hour-long listening sessions—and had administered SSP to dozens of clients. She had experience with all of the SSP Pathways and understood the process well. With a keen interoceptive sense and strong self-awareness, Jill believed she would be safe.

---

* Polyvagal Insight 1: Autonomic State Functions as an Intervening Variable

Her home environment was familiar and comfortable, and she had a close household member checking on her intermittently.

Jill was the lead author of "Combined Delivery Guidelines for EMDR and SSP." She was experienced in creating an individualized SSP delivery plan for each of her clients. She considered all aspects of their situation, including their autonomic tendencies, preferences, the delivery environment, and the other therapeutic modalities they engaged in. Now she did the same preparation for herself.

In her previous SSP usage, she'd had a harder time falling asleep if she listened too late in the day, so she chose to listen first thing in the morning. She set a glass of water and her headphones next to her bed, and each morning upon waking, she drank the water, did some deep breathing, and listened while lying down with her eyes closed. She created a plan for herself to take a break if she noticed increased anxiety or worsening nausea or dizziness. Mindful of such potential dysregulation, she consciously and regularly checked to be sure that continuing was appropriate. With this curiosity and attention as she listened, she found that an hour of listening continued to be safe and appropriate each day.

Jill knew that SSP was not considered a standalone therapy and was often delivered at the same time as other modalities. This knowledge proved valuable on three occasions during this period when she experienced persistent anxiety, brain fog, and a general sense that something was wrong with her brain. From previous experience, she recognized that neurofeedback might provide what her body and brain needed and used it several hours after her SSP listening.

Summary of Provider's Observations about Her Own Response to SSP

After five minutes of listening on the first day, Jill had the new sensation of a sudden physical shift—like an electrical current from her sacrum to the top of her head—that created a better alignment and coherence within her body. After listening for the rest of the hour, her dizziness and brain fog eased and were replaced with a sense of groundedness. When she got up, the ground no longer moved, and she could feel the soles of her feet rooted solidly on the floor.

After listening on the second day, Jill's heart regulated and returned to her normal resting heart rate. She felt relief that her self-intervention was working, and her anxiety lessened.

On the third day, her gastrointestinal symptoms began to resolve. Her interoceptive sense had strengthened from her first round of SSP and that improvement hadn't faded away due to COVID like her sense of taste and smell had. Jill observed that for her and many of her clients, each repetition of SSP Core could generate new benefits. She wondered if that was because the nervous system was strengthened and repatterned in a different way each time.*

On the fourth day, Jill decided to test her memory. Recalling the shock and frustration of being unable to concentrate enough to read and retain information, she cautiously approached a book, hoping for improvement. To her delight, she found herself able to read several chapters, step away, and later recall their contents. This marked a significant milestone, indicating not only a return of some energy and perseverance but also an improvement in her memory.

On the fifth day, her chest congestion started to loosen and her lungs cleared. She tested negative for COVID two days after completing SSP but still had some residual fatigue as well as congestion moving through her lungs. Five days after finishing SSP, Jill was back to teaching an EMDR course, but it took another two months before her senses of taste and smell returned.

In addition to the reduction of symptoms, Jill felt greater balance and flexibility of her ANS, a restored sense of hope, and a reversal of the downward spiral of worry about her health and future.† Being able to care for herself became a powerful antidote to her earlier existential worries.

---

* Polyvagal Insight 7: The ANS Can Be Retuned to Prioritize Connection and Well-Being

† Polyvagal Insight 8: The ANS Is at the Core of Our Physical and Mental Wellness

A Bonus Response to SSP

Five weeks after completing SSP and recovering from most of her COVID symptoms, Jill returned to some personal therapy work she had begun two years before with DBR and AT. She had discontinued her work with these modalities 18 months earlier due to the pandemic, and now she wanted a "tune-up" to address the psychological impacts of being so physically ill. She hoped DBR and AT would help her reprocess the underlying issues that contributed to her anxiety, sense of hopelessness, and anger toward herself and her body.[*]

The AT teacher Jill had worked with previously delivered AT to her, and she separately applied practices from her DBR training on herself. When she first returned to her AT teacher, he noticed a greater openness in her and commented that "a spell has been broken inside of you." Jill herself sensed that something had released, and she had become more present. Similarly, Jill experienced a significant clearing of background activation with DBR.

Jill was aware that after this third round of SSP, she was able to participate in DBR and AT in a way that was radically new for her. She felt no defensiveness, and this allowed her to feel a deeper response. She was "hiding" less from others and from herself. Previously, she had needed to struggle to be really present, but now she found herself totally available.

Looking back, Jill realized she had never truly been herself in the past. She hadn't fully expressed her vulnerabilities or allowed herself to be authentically seen by herself or others, even those closest to her. She began to understand how her "self" had been constructed around and for others. It felt as if she had been hovering around her body, unable to find herself. But after completing SSP and working with AT and DBR, she could now allow herself to be seen and heard. She developed a stronger sense of self and an internal compass. She felt less anger because she no longer felt the need to defend herself. With increased self-compassion, she could care for herself more effectively because she was better attuned

---

* Polyvagal Insight 3: Neuroception Detects Cues of Threat and Safety and Alters Autonomic State

to her bodily state. Reconnecting with her "self" made her feel like she had found her home.

Case Analysis with Dr. Porges

The body's response to COVID includes physical and systemic reactions, with a complex interplay between the immune system and the ANS. We have seen that our foundational survival mechanisms are regulated by the brainstem and expressed in the ANS. Our immune and endocrine systems have a similar role—detecting threats to our survival that are molecular and chemical and reacting by mounting appropriate defenses. If we conceptualize a broader ANS that includes immune and endocrine reactivity, this can allow us to explain the neurophysiological defense reactions we experience when our bodies are invaded by potent pathogens, and the disruptions of our physiological, mental, and behavioral processes that occur in some of us when exposed to COVID.

The polyvagal lens directs a focus on the foundational survival mechanisms regulated by the brainstem and expressed in the ANS, but not exclusively in the ANS. The model positions the ANS as a neural platform for disruptions in physiological, mental, and behavioral processes. In Jill's case, these were inflammation (pain, fatigue, cough, and sore throat); a shutdown of her sensory systems (loss of taste and smell); a gating of her higher cognitive functions (brain fog and working memory problems); and an elevated heart rate. Emotionally, she became anxious and hypervigilant to every symptom.

The acute phase of a viral infection often involves symptoms that signal severe stress to the body that can be interpreted as cues of a serious health threat. These cues typically dissipate along with their physical, mental, and emotional disruptions as one recovers from the acute phase. If acute symptoms persist beyond the initial phase of a viral infection, however, a chronic phase may develop where symptoms become more related to changes in nervous system function (like the cyclic defense loop) and ongoing physiological dysregulation rather than the effects of the original pathogen. This phenomenon is observed in conditions like

Long COVID where individuals may experience prolonged symptoms involving neurological, cognitive, and autonomic disruptions.

Jill's acute phase of COVID resolved before developing into a chronic condition, or Long COVID. Consistent with Jill's experience, though, the SSP provider community has accumulated several reports of SSP supporting a reduction of symptoms associated with COVID and Long COVID.

How SSP Supported Jill's Recovery from COVID

Jill's intuition to wait more than a week before using SSP may have allowed for SSP to be more efficient since it wasn't competing with the acute phase of the illness. By setting up a ritual for daily SSP listening, she was inserting some order and predictability into an otherwise chaotic time.* Taking care of herself allowed for a renewed sense of agency and capacity, something particularly beneficial for one who has experienced trauma.

Jill's system was able to transmit the safety cues embedded in the music of SSP Core through afferent pathways to activate her SES, the nucleus of cranial nerves related to facial expressivity, hearing acuity, vocal prosody, body language, and the vagal influence on heart rate. As these messages accumulated, the ANS could reengage in supporting homeostatic functions in the body and move toward a more optimal state.†

Layers of Healing

Jill's recovery from COVID symptoms and her increased resilience enabled her to turn inward and revisit previous therapeutic modalities, which led to a new and deeper self-understanding. She began to reconcile several aspects of her early life, experiencing these insights in waves. Each new realization enhanced her body awareness, reduced her defensiveness, and deepened her connection with herself and others.

---

* Polyvagal Insight 3: Neuroception Detects Cues of Threat and Safety and Alters Autonomic State

† Polyvagal Insight 2: Autonomic States Bias Our Feelings, Thoughts, and Behaviors

For Jill, each successive experience of SSP deepened her access to a connected ventral state and widened her window of capacity and resilience. She was surprised by her continuous growth. For example, during the case analysis conversation, Jill noticed that she was able to sustain eye contact—it felt good and didn't trigger her previous aversion. Her voice also announced her comfort with its clarity and musicality that resonated as calm and sturdy.[*] As Jill developed new patterns of resilience, she was able to address and discard old patterns that no longer served her. She could now draw people in toward her and give them the gift of accessibility.

The Gift of Accessibility

The nervous system evolved to trust—to be accessible without compromising its stability. And yet, as humans, we tend to become more cautious as we get older, putting up more defenses in new situations. We even raise our children this way—to be vigilant and careful. This is a natural and adaptive response in a world that is not perfectly safe. But in addition to avoiding danger and threat, we also need to find ways to remain open to connection with each other and with new experiences.

A yearning to connect authentically with others is part of our complex, multifaceted evolutionary heritage.[†] Accessibility is a gift. It's a gift that is transformed and magnified in the giving since it is returned many times over—not only to the giver but also to the receiver and the people they connect with.

Violations of predictability and safety, like interrupted early attachment, bullying, abuse, and other forms of exclusion or oppression, cause our nervous system to develop patterns of protection instead of patterns of connection. But even for people who don't appear to have good models of safe relationships in their lives, the mere possibility of accessible and reciprocal relationships can create a burning desire and motivation to feel safe and connected to people. This is why so many people try to

---

[*] Polyvagal Insight 5: Autonomic State Impacts Social Cues

[†] Polyvagal Insight 4: The Power of Social Connection and Co-Regulation

improve their lives and often seek help to do so, whether from therapy, self-help groups, books, or other activities. It may be part of our heritage that when the armor of our defensiveness is let down, a benevolence and love emerge that make life wonderful.

Implications for Daily Life

The COVID pandemic had a devastating impact on many people's health and also had a profound and long-lasting effect on our social engagement and connection. We became attuned to a new threat: the virus. As social beings, we instinctively seek connection when initially faced with a threat. However, the pandemic made us perceive close interactions as dangerous due to potential disease transmission and its consequences.

Our social dynamics shifted. While we experienced a shared global event, it wasn't a unifying one. An invisible pathogen distorted our social bonds in a way that violated our instincts to connect and support one another. Everyone, especially the most vulnerable, became isolated, with effects that persist to this day. But we can work to reestablish our social habits and resume our vital human connections. The sustenance of human connection can be individually life-giving and collectively transformative.

Chapter 16

From Exclusion to Empowerment: A Boy's Journey with Hypermobility Spectrum Disorder

Case Overview

SSP PROVIDER: Njoki Wamae. Contact: njokiwamaetherapy@gmail.com

CLINICAL DISCIPLINE: Njoki is a counselor/psychotherapist grounded in the humanistic approach to psychotherapy and practices in an integrative way. She works with adoptive families and trains teachers and school staff in the social and emotional development of children.

OTHER THERAPEUTIC MODALITIES AND EXPERTISE: Associate lecturer at the Open University; training teachers in the social and emotional development of children, working with adoptive families, and mental health advising and advocacy

CLIENT: Alex (a pseudonym) was 11 years old when Njoki began working with him. He lived in an incredibly loving and supportive household with an older sister who had significant medical needs. Due to psychological and physical threats at school, Alex initially appeared shy and had few social interactions outside of his family.

FEATURES/SYMPTOMS: Hypermobility spectrum disorder (HSD), slow cognitive processing speed and poor working memory, dyslexia, anxiety about starting secondary school, fatigue, hypersensitivities, poor proprioception, urinary incontinence, and frequent accidents related to his hypermobility—several of which were significant and for which he is still monitored at a hospital.

AUTONOMIC TENDENCY: Because of his isolation at school, Alex was stuck in a shutdown dorsal vagal state, but before that, his autonomic tendency was sympathetic with a propensity toward flight more than fight.

ASSESSMENTS: Beyond Njoki's standard intake process and measures, no formal assessments were utilized.

Client Description

As Alex approached the end of primary school (typically ages 5 to 11) and prepared to transition to a larger secondary school (typically ages 11 to 18), his anxiety reached new heights. His apprehension seemed to exceed typical worries associated with transitions and was marked by a profound fear of the unknown. Alex's mother, aware of SSP, hoped it would help him.

When Njoki started working with him, Alex displayed extreme shyness, avoiding eye contact and offering only one-word responses while frequently deferring to his mother for answers. He strongly preferred having his mother present during sessions, which Njoki assured him would be accommodated. He was visibly relieved by this assurance.

The youngest of three siblings, Alex grew up in a nurturing and deeply caring family environment. Having a sister who required extensive medical attention, Alex may have subconsciously prioritized her needs over his own, potentially resulting in a detachment from his personal needs. Furthermore, his history of significant childhood accidents, coupled with ongoing hospital care, underscored the challenges he faced and continued to navigate.

Alex was diagnosed with HSD, a condition characterized by excessive joint flexibility. For Alex, this manifested in clicking joints, intermittent muscle weakness due to loose ligaments and connective tissues, fatigue, pain, gastrointestinal problems, a limited range of dietary choices, and symptoms of autonomic dysfunction.

Alex's SSP Intake Form revealed that, in response to difficult situations, he tended to exhibit sympathetic nervous system reactions such as racing thoughts, increased heart rate, rapid breathing, and focusing difficulty. During these times, Alex responded with constant fidgeting and movement, resisted others' attempts to soothe him, and often resorting to crying or yelling. When overwhelmed, Alex would disengage and withdraw, becoming small and quiet. He lacked the energy to cope and sometimes simply gave in to circumstances, not out of preference but due to feeling too overwhelmed to know what else to do.[*]

Alex exhibited hypersensitivities, particularly in noisy environments where certain volumes and frequencies of sound were uncomfortable for him. Additionally, he occasionally experienced discomfort from bright lights.

Results from Alex's Behavioral Symptoms Test highlighted several areas of concern. These included poor stress tolerance, heightened reactivity to certain sounds, difficulty following instructions, sensory processing challenges, struggles with comprehension in noisy environments, hypervigilance, difficulty relaxing, perseveration of thoughts, and susceptibility to being easily startled.

Another relevant feature is that in safe and trusted environments, such as with his family and close family friends, Alex demonstrated a strong ability to interpret others' emotions, often being the first to do so, especially within his family.

A significant early event in Alex's life was his transition from Lansdowne Primary School to Gladwin Primary School at the age of eight, due to a move to a new house. Leaving behind the familiar and supportive environment of Lansdowne, where he enjoyed good friendships and popularity, was difficult. At Gladwin, Alex found the environment

---

[*] Polyvagal Insight 2: Autonomic States Bias Our Feelings, Thoughts, and Behaviors

markedly different, with a lack of inclusiveness and community, which made it difficult for him to form and maintain friendships. The more welcoming atmosphere of Lansdowne contrasted sharply with his new school's environment, and Alex felt this difference keenly.

Despite these difficulties, it took three years for Alex to confide in his mother about his struggles at his new school and seek support. Once he shared his experience with his parents, they transferred him back to Lansdowne, and Alex was relieved and excited. However, due to COVID-19 and subsequent lockdown measures, Alex was unable to begin immediately at Lansdowne. Instead, he had to continue his education at Gladwin via online learning, which proved to be very challenging and left him feeling sad and stressed. This period marked a turning point for Alex as he began to withdraw, lose confidence, and experience loneliness.

In the autumn term of his last year of primary school (age 11), Alex was finally able to start back at Lansdowne Primary School in person. However, COVID-19 restrictions were still in place, making it difficult for him to rekindle his previous friendships and adjust to the new environment. Despite his natural ability to understand others' emotions, masks and social distancing measures made it difficult for him to interpret social cues.

Additionally, Alex struggled to express his own emotions, possibly because he often prioritized his sister's needs over his own. He also exhibited difficulties with executive functions, including planning and persistence, and he had poor working memory. These challenges led to impulsivity and inflexibility in his behavior.

Prior to the SSP intervention, Alex had had no experience with therapy. His specific goals for SSP included feeling safer, reducing anxiety, and developing a more flexible approach to life. With another school transition approaching, this time to secondary school, and with few friends, Alex's mother was particularly eager for him to establish and maintain meaningful friendships. She hoped that SSP might boost Alex's confidence so that he could engage with life like he did when he felt safe.

SSP Delivery Method

Alex's weekly SSP sessions over 20 weeks were conducted online. He preferred to participate from his bedroom, accompanied by his mother and pet cats.

Njoki started off by teaching Alex about the ANS and helping him to map and understand his own nervous system. The focus was on helping Alex understand that our responses to activation are typically automatic reactions aimed at protecting ourselves from real or perceived threats. To simplify this concept, Njoki utilized Dan Siegel's Hand Model of the Brain (see the glossary).

It was important for Alex to understand his autonomic responses so that he could recognize there were things he could do, with trusted people and on his own, to regulate his emotions. By describing that autonomic reactions are automatic, Njoki aimed to help Alex navigate his resulting emotions without experiencing shame, guilt, or self-blame. She used a story to demonstrate the evolution of the human brain and how we might instinctively fight, flee, freeze, or shut down in threatening situations.

She also used different-sized elastic bands to illustrate his window of capacity and why powering through things, including listening to SSP, was not a good idea. Njoki showed Alex how an overstretched elastic band can snap and cause harm, contrasting it with one that is stretched just enough, which has a greater capacity. With his mother's support, Njoki encouraged Alex to pay attention to his own "elastic" state, helping him recognize his optimal capacity for managing stress and emotions.

Over time, Alex became increasingly interactive and receptive to the information they discussed. They also explored self-care practices together. Alex particularly enjoyed stretching exercises and was proud to teach Njoki one of his favorites. Additionally, he actively participated in deliberate breathing exercises, enjoyed coloring, and eventually felt comfortable sharing his creations with Njoki.

As they began SSP Core, they agreed that Alex did not need to adhere to a specific duration for each session. Instead, they set a maximum limit of 30 minutes per session, allowing Alex the flexibility to listen for any duration between 1 and 30 minutes. This approach empowered Alex to feel a sense of control and choice about his SSP experience. He consistently opted to listen for 15 minutes during each session and navigated the process smoothly.

Each session began with a check-in, where Alex used the descriptors on his autonomic ladder, a tool developed by Deb Dana to help clients become more familiar with their autonomic states,[1] to express how he was feeling. He became increasingly adept at articulating his emotions, sometimes elaborating on why he felt a certain way and other times not. All responses were explicitly welcomed by Njoki. They concluded their sessions by discussing Alex's plans between sessions. Njoki always made a point in the next session to ask about how his plans had unfolded. This fostered a meaningful connection, allowing Alex to link his experiences with sensations in his body. For instance, if he mentioned feeling excited, Njoki would ask how he knew he was excited, prompting him to describe sensations like a lightness in his chest. This practice aimed to help Alex develop awareness of his bodily sensations and their meanings.

Alex's mum joined him in the room during their sessions, and they positioned themselves so Njoki could see both of them. One of the most heartwarming aspects of their interaction was a coordinated dance they shared, gently mirroring the tender connection between a mother and her baby. Alex's mum intuitively provided support whenever Alex needed a check-in, always present and exchanging smiles with him whenever he glanced her way. This lovely dynamic unfolded at every session, and Njoki cherished the opportunity to witness their special bond. Additionally, Alex's mum demonstrated deep respect for his boundaries and autonomy, only engaging further when invited, whether verbally or through nonverbal cues.

Alex's two kittens also played a significant role in their sessions, enhancing their connection by providing a safe and enjoyable topic of conversation for him. As their sessions progressed, typically by mid-hour, Alex would adjust his camera to show Njoki where his kittens were resting. Occasionally, he would even cuddle or stroke his kitten, Jiji, who was the more agreeable one.

Summary of Provider's Observations about the Client's Response to SSP

Alex experienced very encouraging responses to SSP. Even though he was not quite able to describe the changes that had occurred, his behavior told it all. Njoki and his mother noticed a clear improvement in his confidence levels, as well as a greater sense of flexibility and happiness.

Prior to SSP, Alex had been dealing with instances of banter that bordered on bullying behavior at school. This clashed with his gentle, loving, and considerate traits. To protect himself, he became wary of social interactions, which left him feeling somewhat isolated.

Following SSP, Alex became more confident, possibly having learned to discern cues of safety and threat more accurately. His mum reported an exciting milestone: for the first time in a long time, Alex brought a friend from school home. He was eager for his friend to meet his kittens, a clear sign of his newfound confidence and willingness to engage socially. This visit was a joyous and positive experience for Alex and his family.

Another remarkable aspect of Alex's journey was his involvement in theater. Initially, he auditioned for a local theater group with modest expectations, aiming for a minor role where he could blend into the background. However, after the SSP sessions, Alex's confidence grew, and he decided to audition for a more prominent role. His mother expressed her delight, saying, "I am very pleased that Alex is stretching himself and is interested in these things."

In the UK, children in Year 6, typically ages 10 to 11, are generally allowed to travel on buses independently as a way to prepare for secondary school journeys. Most children embrace this newfound freedom with excitement and enjoy riding the bus. Before SSP, Alex would not have considered taking the bus alone and felt apprehensive about navigating noisy and crowded places like shops. However, after SSP, Alex successfully took a bus to his local shopping center and even ventured into several shops, engaging in browsing—a feat previously unimaginable for him. This newfound independence was a cause for celebration for his family, marking another remarkable change facilitated by SSP.

Summary of Client's Mother's Reflections on Client's Response to SSP

Alex derived many benefits from SSP. His anxiety decreased while his confidence increased, leading to the blossoming of his SES and the exploration of new opportunities and experiences. He formed new friendships, and when his mum asked him if he thought SSP had helped him, Alex responded, "It gave me the push to do things." He also thought his memory had improved, and he felt more confident and able to find a more compatible friend group.

His sensory sensitivities decreased, enabling him to tolerate background noise better and explore new foods. This change enhanced his dining experience in noisy pubs with his family and enabled him to participate in a musical production, despite its loudness. After SSP, Alex demonstrated more initiative in pursuing activities aligned with his interests and stretching himself to achieve his goals. He expressed interest in repeating SSP and, in the meantime, he curated his own calming music playlist.

When Alex changed primary schools, he experienced a disconnection from his previous friends for approximately three to five years. However, after SSP, Alex reached out to an old friend and successfully reestablished their relationship. Things progressed smoothly, leading to Alex having a sleepover with the friend. He also became more open, attending birthday parties and immersing himself in the festivities with enjoyment. These were significant milestones for Alex, marking the reemergence of a happy and confident young person.

Case Analysis with Dr. Porges

HSD represents a broad spectrum of conditions, such as Ehlers Danlos syndrome, characterized by joint hypermobility. Individuals with HSD often experience systemic symptoms such as gastrointestinal issues, autonomic dysregulation, and emotional and musculoskeletal problems.

Dysautonomia, or dysregulation of the ANS, was identified in 63 percent of subjects with HSD in a recent study.[2] Some individuals with a genetic predisposition to HSD remain asymptomatic until triggered by a trauma, such as a car accident. This trauma can cause the ANS to retune and lock into a state of defense, providing the neurophysiological platform for various behavioral, physiological, and psychological symptoms to be expressed. Hypothetically, the autonomic and emotional symptoms may not be part of the genetic program of HSD but are piggybacked onto a common trigger of threat. Thus, optimistically, the symptoms dependent on autonomic state, such as emotional regulation, might be managed through interventions like SSP, which retune the ANS. Consistent with this hypothesis, Alex's symptoms, including hypersensitivities, anxiety, gastrointestinal issues, and fatigue, were influenced by autonomic dysregulation.

Hypersensitivities

Alex had significant hypersensitivities to sound, light, and certain foods linked to a hypervigilant nervous system. These included his heightened sensitivity to others' emotions. In a defensive state, Alex's body detected even the slightest cues, keeping him constantly alert and watchful. After undergoing SSP, his body could access a calm ventral vagal state, allowing these hypersensitivities to subside. Consequently, he could tolerate the noise at pubs and theaters, and bright lights became less problematic. He also began experimenting with a wider range of foods.

Anxiety

Heightened anxiety, common in autonomic dysregulation, is part of a cycle and can seem like both a cause and a result of a nervous system stuck in a state of threat. The ANS adaptively responds by increasing heart rate, blood pressure, and breathing rate and releasing stress hormones, the effect of which is to cause sensations that can increase feelings of anxiety and therefore continue the cycle.

Because it is metabolically costly, heightened anxiety would eventually exhaust Alex's nervous system, causing it to shift into a dorsal vagal state, making him seem withdrawn and shy. Alex thus oscillated between sympathetic and dorsal states during challenging times at school. However, after SSP, Alex was able to break free from this cyclic defense loop and access his calm and connected ventral vagal state. It was then that Alex's authentic self began to show.

Gastrointestinal Issues

Being trapped in the cyclic defense loop can significantly affect gut function, leading to various symptoms such as constipation (from sympathetic activation), diarrhea (from dorsal vagal shutdown), and nausea and vomiting due to delayed stomach emptying (gastroparesis). These disruptions can lead to abnormal gut function, including poor nutrient absorption, bacterial overgrowth, and overall pain or discomfort. After SSP, Alex's ANS was no longer stuck in a defense mode, allowing his gut to heal and his symptoms to abate. As his vomiting and tummy aches reduced, he was able to expand his diet.

Fatigue

Alex suffered from painful joints, and the pain itself was exhausting. Being stuck in a cyclic defense loop made daily activities even more taxing, worsening his persistent fatigue. Anxiety, digestive problems, and poor sleep further drained his energy. However, when his nervous system was retuned through SSP, his autonomic functions stabilized, resolving his sleep issues, anxiety, and digestive problems. As a result, his energy returned, allowing him to enjoy social interactions and pursue his interests with renewed enthusiasm.

Psychoeducation

Njoki was intentional about creating a safe and trusting relationship with Alex, carefully attuning to his needs and teaching him about his nervous system. This connection allowed Alex to open up about his experiences and the changes he was going through. Njoki introduced a shared language by using a rubber band as a metaphor for Alex's nervous system, often asking him if he felt loose or tight. At times, he described his "rubber band" as so tight that it felt like it might snap. Njoki explained that by paying attention to his "rubber band," he could better recognize his autonomic states and know when to pull back from stressors. The metaphor became a practical tool he could use in his everyday life.

Fitting In

Several aspects of Alex's life that are simply part of who he is—his periodic incontinence, accidents due to his HSD, and his mixed-race background—were more noticeable at his new school. Additionally, having just moved to a new house and started a new school, Alex experienced multiple significant changes simultaneously, which felt unfamiliar and therefore unsafe. His hypersensitivities also heightened his awareness of the feelings and reactions of everyone around him.

Alex may have experienced his racial identity as different for the first time at age nine when he switched schools. His previous school, Lansdowne, was more diverse, while Gladwin was less so. In a predominantly single-race community like Gladwin, racial differences can stand out more. Children at Alex's age just want to fit in with their peers and to feel they belong and are valued. Every little thing that doesn't conform— from clothing to hair to what's on or even in their lunchbox—can be magnified. This is especially true for people who are hypersensitive to their environment, making it even more important to feel validated.

Alex was dealing with much more than his parents realized. Feeling different in a way that deeply matters poses a significant threat to the ANS. When this difference pertains to a person's core identity rather than something superficial, it creates an ongoing threat that can keep the ANS in a prolonged defensive state. Alex's ability to navigate this challenge was largely due to the unwavering support and love he received from his family.

SSP also helped. His mum observed a noticeable change in Alex's demeanor after SSP: he felt less concerned about "sticking out." This newfound confidence was evident in his willingness to audition for a larger role in the school production, try new experiences, and be more authentically himself.

Results

When asked, Alex wasn't sure SSP had a significant impact. It's common for clients, especially children and adolescents, to be less aware of their changes. Since the changes are spontaneous and not intentional, they often occur without awareness. The changes shift into awareness when others respond differently. Sensitive and explicit feedback may reframe the individual's sense of self and, if appropriate, can provide helpful encouragement. In Alex's case, people around him noticed spontaneous social engagement, increased confidence, a lighter demeanor, and greater comfort being himself. His anxiety reduced significantly, and he began trying new things like inviting friends over, taking the bus by himself, and creating his own calming playlist. As his behavior and autonomic state changed, his social network expanded as others spontaneously responded to him being more accessible.

Implications for Daily Life

A sense of belonging is a meaningful input to our nervous system, providing predictability that helps us feel safe and connected. Being part of a community where we feel included and valued offers a stable support network essential for emotional growth. When we feel like we belong, we become more flexible, curious, and socially engaged, which helps us navigate social interactions with greater confidence and ease. This creates a positive feedback loop, fostering creativity and exploration and allowing us to be our authentic selves rather than feeling judged or pressured to conform. Furthermore, a strong sense of belonging can reduce uncertainty, offer reliable co-regulation, decrease anxiety and depression, enhance overall well-being, and make it easier to face challenges.

Chapter 17

The Importance of "Being" Rather Than "Doing" as an SSP Provider

Case Overview

SSP PROVIDER: Paula Scatoloni, LCSW, SEP. Website: paulascatoloni.com/about/

CLINICAL DISCIPLINE: Paula is a practitioner, guide, speaker, and contemporary sound healer specializing in somatics, movement, and the therapeutic use of sound to support healing in the individual and collective nervous system. She is the lead author of "Combined Delivery Guidelines for Somatic Experiencing and Safe and Sound Protocol (SSP)."

OTHER THERAPEUTIC MODALITIES AND EXPERTISE: Interpersonal neurobiology, PVT, Somatic Experiencing, Bodywork and Somatic Education, Transforming the Experienced-Based Brain, Sensorimotor Psychotherapy, Body-Mind Centering, Embodied Recovery, Biofield Tuning, and spiritual wisdom teachings

CLIENT: David (a pseudonym) is a somatic therapist whose modalities include Rolfing Structural Integration, Somatic Experiencing, expressive arts therapy, and SSP. He is also a mental health counselor and has training in Somatic Resilience and Regulation with Kathy Kain and Stephen Terrell. He approached Paula for experiential training in SSP delivery.

FEATURES/SYMPTOMS: Paula teaches her SSP delivery approach to other clinicians by offering a comprehensive and immersive experience of SSP. David's work with her was for personal and professional growth rather than targeting specific features or symptoms. Instead, they both anticipated an organic unfolding of information as the SSP sessions progressed.

AUTONOMIC TENDENCY: David's nervous system had not developed optimal ventral capacity or what would be referred to as foundational regulation.[1] As such, it had been shaped to manage sympathetic arousal with a dorsal response. This is often referred to as a "functional freeze" in somatic terms describing his ability to engage in basic life tasks while in a "freeze," or blended, state of sympathetic and dorsal physiology.

ASSESSMENTS: No formal assessments were utilized. Paula used what she learned about David as they worked together to develop a picture of his attachment dynamics,[2] and from there she began to assist in the reshaping of his ANS.

Client Description

As a longtime, skilled practitioner of Rolfing Structural Integration, David had developed a deep understanding of the body, movement, and awareness. Building on this foundation, he pursued a certification in Somatic Experiencing through which he delved into PVT. This exploration not only clarified many concepts for David personally but also enriched his therapeutic work with clients. This motivated him to explore SSP further.

David had done SSP for the first time on his own, and his deep attunement to his own bodily reactions enhanced his awareness of physiological state changes. He could tell that SSP was improving his nervous system regulation. He also understood that it was a relational tool, and he was interested in experiencing it with a "present other" for a more co-regulatory experience. Eager to learn more about how another Somatic Experiencing Practitioner used it in their practice, he reached out to Paula, who had assisted in his Somatic Experiencing training and clinical consultations.

In addition to his intention to learn more about SSP delivery, David was curious about how SSP might change his relationship dynamics.

SSP Delivery Method

According to Paula, "Sound is medicine." She emphasizes that sound and vibration create powerful effects on clients' physiology, psychology, and emotional well-being, enabling them to access more of their innate human capacity. Paula uses SSP to harness this therapeutic potential. A key factor in unlocking SSP's efficacy is the provider's embodiment and what Thomas Hübl terms "attuned relational presence."[3] Paula provides experiential learning for SSP providers to cultivate and deepen this quality, elevating SSP delivery to enrich clients' experiences.

An essential element of Paula's approach to SSP delivery is enhancing her client's embodiment by exploring their relational templates. Drawing from her studies with Bonnie Bainbridge Cohen,[4] Paula understands how early relational experiences shape the nervous system to orient toward safety or fear. She recognizes the influence of environmental, social, and cultural factors in shaping these tendencies and how they affect an individual's engagement in the developmental relational movements outlined by Cohen: yield (finding rest in relational safety), push (cultivating self-awareness through proprioception and interoception to support healthy boundaries), reach (expanding beyond familiar boundaries to follow curiosity), and grasp and pull (strengthening capacity for deeper intimacy with others and the world).

Paula incorporates Cohen's developmental relational movements into the SSP listening process to help her clients transition from rigidity to flow. She creates a somatic experience of safe relational yielding for her clients by using pillows, blankets, and supports positioned around their bodies. Paula likens this to the comforting environment of an infant resting in a crib, where signals of comfort and safety are abundant.

Throughout David's SSP sessions, Paula carefully observed the emergence of developmental movements and provided feedback to help him track his growth.

Being embodied and present with her clients is essential to Paula. She believes that when clients feel deeply met on physical, emotional, and energetic levels, parts of themselves that have been dissociated or disowned begin to surface. Paula encourages her clients to notice and become aware of any physical, emotional, mental, or somatic reactions that arise during their SSP listening. This awareness aids in digesting and integrating these responses into the nervous system.

Focusing on repatterning the early relational template, Paula takes time with clients to identify their adaptive strategies either before or during the SSP listening process. With nervous system support provided by both SSP and her embodied presence, clients' adaptive strategies begin to soften, allowing space for their more desirable strategies to emerge.

Paula paces SSP sessions to allow each element that arises in the listening ample time to integrate. Thus, the sessions are scheduled once per week. If a difficult early experience surfaces during SSP, clients can bring this material to their individual therapist to process in detail before the next listening session.

When Paula offers SSP in a group format for providers and individuals, she typically divides the listening into 10-minute increments. At each pause, clients focus on their sensations, emotions, thoughts, images, and behaviors.

Given David's extensive background in somatic therapy, Paula allowed him to decide whether to pause the music when something needed processing. Typically, she guided him to observe his reactions with curiosity and to use mindful awareness and self-compassion as he engaged with emerging aspects of himself. During their weekly sessions, David's listening times ranged from 10 to 30 minutes, depending on what arose. Approaching the experience as a learning process, David also discussed clients and SSP usage with Paula. Overall, his experience of listening, learning, and processing spanned six months.

Summary of Provider's Observations about the Client's Response to SSP

David's ability to track his own internal system facilitated a smooth and effortless interaction with Paula. There was a steady ebb and flow during the listening process, providing ample time for both his internal processing and his questions. As a Somatic Experiencing Practitioner, Paula was also adept at observing subtle nuances occurring and guiding his attention to them when necessary.

As David became more aware of his defensive structures, he gained a deeper understanding of them and explored them through his developmental movements while listening to SSP. Outside the sessions, he observed that he was better able to stay embodied and connect with others. Additionally, he found himself less reliant on food for regulation and more capable of accessing internal sources for balance. His ability to identify his needs (push), express them (reach), and accept relational support (grasp and pull) began to shift positively.

As David's comfort with himself grew, he experienced less social or relational awkwardness. By staying present in his "self," he began to monitor his hunger and exercise needs more effectively. These were not data points for him in the beginning, but when the shifts started to emerge and his interoception strengthened, he became more attuned to them. He shifted from accommodating others to focusing on his own needs in the moment. When we feel safe, we use our energy differently; we absorb others' energy less and our boundaries become more distinct.*

David was now able to ask for what he needed and confidently say no when something didn't align with his goals or availability. Over the six months, his exploration of various aspects of himself enhanced his ability to discern and set his boundaries, identify and express emotions, and experience increased intimacy with others.

---

* Polyvagal Insight 3: Neuroception Detects Cues of Threat and Safety and Alters Autonomic State

Paula and David worked together to enhance his ability to access more of his authentic self. They focused on his internal sensations during the listening process to develop his proprioception and interoception. This approach helped him reconnect with his true essence, often referred to as his "self"—the part of him connected to his early years and his true identity. In one session, David used a blank page and colored pencils to create art as he listened. This creative process brought him a deeper awareness of his childhood connection to art and its link to his creativity or "spiritual essence."

David became more embodied in himself as he experienced increasing safety through the SSP process with Paula. As David's capacity to perceive relational support as accessible and nonthreatening grew, he was able to more easily yield to relational safety in the present moment. This shift allowed him to interact with his clients from a place of "being" rather than "doing." Paula emphasized to her clients that the provider's ability to embody this attuned relational presence was crucial. This approach created an environment of interpersonal safety that enhanced the healing effects of SSP.*

Summary of Client's Reflections on Their Response to SSP

Since his experience of SSP with Paula, David has found it easier to identify and express his needs in relationships and set appropriate boundaries without fearing loss of connection. He now feels more comfortable reaching out for support rather than feeling he must handle challenges alone. As a result, he relies less on self-regulation and more on co-regulation with others.

David, who had previously operated from an "anxious relational strategy" and tended to appease others to maintain connections, found significant changes after completing SSP with Paula. He engaged in less appeasement and became more attuned to his own needs. With greater presence and awareness, David could choose whether to follow his

---

* Polyvagal Insight 4: The Power of Social Connection and Co-Regulation

"well-worn pattern" of accommodating others or to decide for himself in the moment whether to make himself available. He experienced this change as an "unblending" of the younger parts of himself that had set aside his own needs for others while growing up. David noted that when he chose to help now, it came from a more genuine place. He reported a sense of integration and a "new normal" in his interpersonal patterns.

Paula encouraged David to tune in to his interoceptive cues between sessions. He discovered that he was a highly sensitive person who had developed a method of overriding this sensitivity to function effectively in the world. With Paula's support, he learned to pause and explore his sensitivity during the SSP process. By working with it as a resource, he was able to find the "just right" level of connection with others and the world on any given day. He observed his state shifting from sympathetic activation and functional freeze to a ventral vagal state, allowing these processes to unfold naturally. This exploration also facilitated the integration of implicit memories, enabling him to create a new narrative around specific life events.

As David's self-awareness and nervous system capacity grew, he spent less time in defensive states and noticed improvements in his executive functioning. As he moved away from his functional freeze tendency, he found he was masking less in his relationships.* He accepted that he experienced himself as neurodivergent and found a great sense of relief in realizing that he didn't need to conform to neurotypical standards.

David achieved a deeper level of foundational regulation through the SSP listening process. He learned to access this state more consistently and continued to shape his nervous system to maintain it regularly. This transformation positively influenced his perspectives and relationships with others, including his clients.†

He was aware of some sadness when reflecting on his previous strategies of "overdoing" in a relationship. However, he approached himself

---

* Polyvagal Insight 7: The ANS Can Be Retuned to Prioritize Connection and Well-Being

† Polyvagal Insight 1: Autonomic State Functions as an Intervening Variable

with compassion and understanding and supported this aspect of self by engaging in relationships in a more balanced way.

David also became better able to use SSP to deepen his clients' capacity for embodiment. He recognized that his attuned relational presence[*] greatly enhanced the effectiveness of SSP delivery. By being more present and attuned, he helped his clients connect more deeply with their embodied experiences and achieve greater benefits from SSP.

Case Analysis with Dr. Porges

The role of the SSP provider is crucial, as SSP is a potent intervention, particularly when delivered in an attuned and embodied way. This is especially clear in this case, where the client was also a Somatic Experiencing Practitioner and SSP provider. Paula and David's symbiotic relationship, use of common treatment modalities and training, and shared language gave the experience a feeling of ease and understanding.

Showing up in the most attuned and embodied way is vital because the accessibility of the provider's nervous system is an important prerequisite for the music. Designed to be experienced alongside an attuned provider or loving parent, SSP is most effective when the cues of safety in the music are amplified by safety and co-regulation from another. SSP provides signals of safety to the nervous system and an invitation for connection. Without this connection, the nervous system might interpret the signals as threats. By receiving SSP from Paula, David was able to heal in connection, and he became more embodied and connected both within himself and with others.

Experiencing the Value of "Being" Rather Than "Doing"

David learned from Paula's attuned relational presence that, as a provider, the key is to let go of any pressure to do more than simply be present and attuned with the client. Just being with them, without any demands or expectations, is more impactful than any doing. The provider's authentic presence and attentive witnessing are the most therapeutic intervention.

---

[*] Polyvagal Insight 5: Autonomic State Impacts Social Cues

The safer people feel—regardless of their professional background—the more authentically they can engage and express themselves. Memories and vulnerabilities may surface naturally and in their own time, underscoring the importance of not rushing the process. When physiological or psychological reactions arise, they present an opportunity to pause and address them. David felt secure enough with Paula to explore and integrate any issues that emerged, enabling him to access insights and experiences that had previously been out of reach in other therapeutic settings.

There was a symmetry in the relationship between David and Paula that was very beneficial. Paula could be with and witness David without imposing any expectations or demands, which alleviated any pressure on David to meet her needs or fulfill certain expectations. In many aspects of life, such as parenting, education, and in our culture generally, there is often a tendency to "fix" problems. However, what people truly need is someone who can validate their experiences without trying to impose solutions. Paula excelled in providing this kind of supportive presence rather than taking on the role of a fixer.

This approach shifted David's perspective on SSP from a self-regulatory tool to a co-regulatory one. While he could listen to SSP on his own, he preferred to listen alongside Paula, as the shared experience offered him significantly more. The co-regulation with Paula was instrumental in facilitating meaningful change. Through their collaborative sessions, David became aware of aspects of himself that had previously eluded him.

David found that SSP with Paula enhanced an authentic communication of his needs. He now felt safe enough in his relationships to be in disagreement without feeling compelled to appease as had been his pattern. SSP helped to interrupt that pattern. Retuning the ANS so we can feel safe enough to be who we truly are is the aim of SSP.

Supportive Elements of SSP Delivery

Several elements enhance the SSP experience by providing structure and creating the time and space needed for evolution and integration.

By having many tools, techniques, and approaches, SSP providers can customize the most effective strategy for each client. Some of the strategies that Paula and David employed are described below.

Being an Attuned Provider

Paula's genuine presence and attentive witnessing of David's experience allowed him to relax and be his authentic self. When vulnerabilities and defensive reactions are witnessed, they can often diminish or even disappear.

Including Curiosity

Curiosity is a critical feature that puts space between the reaction (neuroception) and the interpretation (feeling) of interoception by higher (conscious) brain structures.

Listening at a Slow Pace

Meeting weekly and listening for just 10 or more minutes during the session allowed for better integration, more practice with interoception, and greater access to David's emotions. Going slowly gave him the chance to practice a new awareness in the world between the weekly sessions and the ability to slowly integrate what arose for processing. Focusing on interoceptive cues in the weeks between sessions was very supportive. He experienced a restoration of his interoception, which allowed for better awareness of his emotions and thought patterns.

Incorporating Creative Art

New insights can emerge when listening while doing something creative. David became more open and available when he drew freestyle and especially so when he drew with his nondominant hand. This seemed to give him access to a different mindset.

Using Movement

Paula incorporated somatic additions related to the developmental movements of grasp and push. David used grasp by holding an object while listening to add sensory input, and he explored push by practicing assertiveness in relationships. Both movements were evocative and reparative.

Paula finds that if fear or anxiety arises, these developmental movements can temper that.

Introducing light movement into SSP delivery can help people stay more regulated and present. Fun and playful movement can stimulate the ventral vagal complex and reduce both sympathetic activation and dorsal shutdown. However, overly vigorous movement may shift clients from a ventral vagal state to sympathetic activation.

SSP for SSP Providers

SSP providers deserve the same nurturing care they give to others. Maintaining a ventral vagal state is crucial for their effectiveness, as it enhances the SSP experience for their clients. When providers are fully present and attuned, SSP becomes significantly more impactful, creating a ripple effect that benefits not only the client but also their family, community, and beyond.

Implications for Daily Life

Our autonomic state shapes our physical, mental, and emotional experiences, influencing how we engage with the world and impacting those around us. When we are regulated and offer "attuned relational presence," we enhance our availability to others, fostering co-regulation and enabling genuine, meaningful connections.

There are times when we need co-regulation ourselves, seeking empathy and support from others. Experiencing this mutual support can be one of life's greatest joys, creating a shared sense of safety. Operating from this place of safety allows everything to flow more smoothly, helping us express care, joy, and authenticity with ease.

Conclusion

When scientific theory and clinical practice come together as they did with SSP, they combine different perspectives and expertise, which improve the quality and range of both research and client care. This teamwork helps turn scientific discoveries into practical treatments, allowing clinicians and scientists to make a real difference.

With the collaboration of SSP providers, new ideas and creativity emerged, leading to better outcomes. New approaches were developed that benefited clients and also have provided a new lens for providers to work with them. As a new tool and approach, SSP has not only improved client results but has also kept providers, scientists, and researchers motivated to learn and innovate further.

Writing this book has reminded the authors of the amazing insights from the community of SSP providers. Listening and learning from providers and their clients has been incredible. Their stories of change illustrate how SSP works.

Unlike medication, SSP's impact depends on the relationship between provider and client. The best outcomes occur when there's a trusting connection, allowing the client to relax and explore their feelings without being triggered by past associations. The neural basis for this trust lies in the ventral vagal complex in the brainstem, which supports social engagement and co-regulation. SSP was designed to activate this system, making the ANS calm and incompatible with defensive behaviors.

The ventral vagal complex, part of the SES, is ready at birth to help coordinate sucking, swallowing, and breathing while signaling needs through vocalizations. As the individual matures, this system helps them communicate socially and engage in reciprocal interactions, leading to co-regulation. When a baby is calm, it sends positive signals to the caregiver's nervous system, creating a calming cycle. Conversely, a fussy baby can disrupt the caregiver's nervous system. PVT highlights the ventral vagal complex's role in fostering trust and co-regulation beyond basic needs. SSP was designed to activate this system, promoting social engagement instead of defense. Thus, SSP helps us navigate the world more effectively by enhancing natural social engagement abilities.

Although each story in the book is unique, there are common themes. First, the client feels "safe enough" to experience SSP. Second, even if SSP temporarily disrupts their behavior, the strong relationship with the provider helps them process and overcome this disruption. Third, completing the SSP protocol makes their nervous system more flexible, resilient, and better at engaging with others. Perhaps the most significant change is the increased ability to co-regulate with others, expressed as playfulness, curiosity, and trust.

The clinical applications of SSP document the power of acoustic signals of safety when delivered in a safe, trusting context. The intervention's name highlights that safety is essential for the nervous system to retune and respond. Successful outcomes return the nervous system to its natural state, which can detect threats but also become curious to explore, be flexible, and resilient when supported by safe relationships.

We learned that co-regulation and accessibility are as contagious as fear and hate, but they emerge from different physiological states. Co-regulation makes people feel safe, promoting health, growth, and social engagement. Understanding how being stuck in a threat state limits connection and quality of life has served as a motivation to develop and apply SSP as a technique to retune the nervous system toward co-regulation and compassion.

Throughout the writing of this book, the authors have truly appreciated the providers and clients sharing their experiences. Learning from them has been invaluable in integrating theory with real-world experiences. Seeing SSP evolve and make a difference in so many lives has been a profoundly gratifying and fulfilling experience.

Acknowledgments

From the Coauthors

Steve and Karen extend their profound appreciation to the SSP providers and clients who shared their stories for the case studies and vignettes. We are deeply moved by your generosity of spirit, skill, curiosity, and resilience. Getting to know you and your experiences has been an honor. Your contributions will enrich the SSP knowledge base, inspire fellow clinicians, and offer hope to future clients.

We offer our gratitude to the wonderful team at Sounds True, especially Anastasia Pellouchoud, Angela Wix, and Leslie Brown for their advocacy and meticulous attention to the manuscript. Their efforts ensured it conveys the possibilities for connection and change through PVT and SSP in a clear and sensitive way. We also thank our foreign publishers and translators for bringing this book to a broader, international audience.

Thank you also to Lisa Gleeson and Jerry Mocciola for their creativity and care in producing the charts, figures, and videos featured in the book. Lastly, we extend our appreciation to our colleagues who contributed video demonstrations of practices and activities for nervous system regulation: Rebecca Bailey, Linda Chamberlain, Deb Dana, Amber Gray, Jill Miller, Betsy Polatin, Arielle Schwartz, Donnalea Van Vleet Goeltz, and Jan Winhall.

From Steve

I would like to extend my deepest gratitude to several individuals whose contributions have been crucial to the realization and success of both this book and SSP.

Firstly, I want to acknowledge Karen Onderko, whose role has been indispensable in formulating the structure and implementing the content of our book. Karen's contributions enabled the insights gained from the application of SSP to be conveyed in words. It has been through her compassionate connections with providers and clients that their rich personal narratives have been crafted to convey the transformative power of SSP. Even more foundational, Karen's dedication has been pivotal in transitioning SSP from laboratory research into an accessible clinical product. As Integrated Listening Systems (iLs) licensed the technology, Karen took on the role of SSP's guardian, guiding its early development and integration within iLs. The emails we began receiving, detailing SSP's profound impact, inspired us to consider compiling these insights into a book. This work reflects not only our collaboration but Karen's invaluable contributions to the development and the successful application of SSP.

I also wish to thank Randall Redfield, who, as CEO of iLs, played a critical role in supporting SSP. Randall's backing, alongside Karen's efforts, was fundamental in evolving the technology into a widely accessible therapeutic tool used by thousands.

A special mention goes to Jason Tafler and the Unyte Health team. After iLs was acquired by Unyte Health in 2019, Jason expanded SSP's reach through the development of a remote app delivery system and a broader provider network, enhancing SSP's accessibility and impact.

The transformation of SSP from a theoretical concept into a practical treatment owes much to the shared experiences of those who embraced it. Their narratives underscore how PVT provides a compassionate framework for understanding nervous system responses and recovery.

I am also grateful to the innovative SSP providers who have extended its applications into psychotherapy, medicine, education, and performance, demonstrating its potential to enhance social engagement and autonomic regulation.

Lastly, I want to acknowledge my wife, Sue Carter, whose pioneering research on oxytocin and social bonds has greatly influenced my work. Sue's support and intellectual curiosity have been invaluable, as have the contributions of our sons, Seth and Eric. Seth coauthored "Our Polyvagal World: How Safety and Trauma Change Us," and Eric is exploring vagal stimulation for PTSD relief. In addition, our sons served as pilot subjects as I developed the technology embedded in SSP. Their involvement reflects our family's commitment to understanding the biology of trust and connection.

From Karen

I am deeply grateful to Steve Porges for the opportunity to work with and learn from him over the past nine years. This book is a testament to our rewarding collaboration.

My heartfelt thanks and love go to my husband, Bob Doherty, my daughters, Evan, Jane, and Camille, and my family and friends. Your encouragement has been a steady source of support throughout this fascinating journey.

I have immense gratitude for the valued input and support from the following people: Rebecca Bailey and Jaycee Dugard for their insights into appeasement and fawn; Liz Charles for her steadfast friendship, time, and collaboration—her considerable medical and clinical knowledge has been invaluable; Sharon Cravitz for her insightful observations on PVT from her perspective as an outside observer; Dara Hoffman Fox for their guidance on respectful language related to gender identity; Caryn Mirriam Goldberg for her incisive writing advice and coaching; Teresa Hommel for her careful editing and the inspiring personal feedback she offered on the material; Heidi Juniper for her exuberant co-regulation; Megan Mackay for her valuable advice on writing sensitively about autism; Emily Reaser for generously offering a lovely environment for distraction-free writing; Carrie Strauch for numerous conversations that clarified my thinking; and George Thompson for his guidance and timely help when I needed it most.

Lastly, I'm grateful for SSP. Listening to SSP Balance while writing helped me stay regulated and productive.

Appendix 1

Assessment Descriptions

Autonomic Resilience Screener

The Autonomic Resilience Screener (ANS Screener) is a subjective questionnaire developed by a group of SSP providers aiming for an efficient tool to gain insights into their clients' ANS in a comprehensive and inviting manner. The screener comprises six sections: emotions, body, sensory, behavior, cognitive, and social. This tool is designed to bring clinical attention to relevant experiences during SSP delivery, facilitating the process of delivery, titration, response tracking, and change measuring post-SSP.

Behavior Assessment System for Children

The Behavior Assessment System for Children third edition (BASC-3) is a comprehensive set of standardized, norm-referenced tools designed to assess the behavior and emotional functioning of children and adolescents. The BASC-3 is widely used in educational, clinical, and research settings to identify behavioral and emotional challenges, assess treatment progress, and inform goal setting and treatment planning.

Body Perception Questionnaire Autonomic Symptoms Scale

The Body Perception Questionnaire Autonomic Symptoms Scale (BPQ20-ANS) is a standardized self-report questionnaire that assesses the frequency of specific body stress reactions in organs that are innervated by the ANS. Though each unique part of the body may have its own reason for activation, the parts are linked by the ANS, a brain-body network that responds to everyday stress. Combined scores from organs throughout the body provide a measure of autonomic stress response patterns. The questionnaire has been used in a range of international neural, behavioral, and clinical studies and translated into more than a dozen languages and has been corroborated with sensor-based measures of autonomic function assessed at the laboratory at Indiana University.[1] The BPQ20-ANS is available from the Traumatic Stress Research Consortium at Indiana University (traumascience.org/body-perception-questionnaire).

Brain-Body Center Sensory Scales

The Brain-Body Center Sensory Scales (BBCSS) is a self-report questionnaire based on PVT that links cranial nerve feedback and regulatory mechanisms to behavior. The adult and child versions include questions across four subscales: auditory processing, visual processing, tactile processing, and eating and feeding behaviors. More information is available from the Traumatic Stress Research Consortium at Indiana University (traumascience.org/bbcss-self-scoring-form).

Hospital Anxiety and Depression Scale

The Hospital Anxiety and Depression Scale (HADS) was developed as a self-assessment scale for detecting states of depression and anxiety in people who are receiving medical treatment. It consists of 14 items, divided into two subscales: one for anxiety symptoms and one for depression symptoms. The HADS is widely used in clinical settings to screen for anxiety and depression among patients with physical illnesses.

Minnesota Multiphasic Personality Inventory-2

The Minnesota Multiphasic Personality Inventory-2 (MMPI-2) is a widely used psychological assessment tool that measures various aspects of an individual's personality and psychopathology. It is designed to assist in the diagnosis, treatment planning, and research of mental health conditions.

Parkinson's Disease Questionnaire

The Parkinson's Disease Questionnaire (PDQ-39) is a widely used self-report assessment tool designed to measure the health-related quality of life in individuals with Parkinson's disease. It evaluates various aspects of daily functioning, emotional well-being, and social interaction that may be affected by the condition.

Patient Health Questionnaire-9

The Patient Health Questionnaire-9 (PHQ) is a self-assessment tool used to screen and assess the severity of depression symptoms.

Pediatric Symptom Checklist

The Pediatric Symptom Checklist (PSC) is a brief, standardized tool designed to screen for emotional, behavioral, and cognitive issues in children and adolescents. It consists of questions that address emotional and behavioral concerns, attention problems, and social difficulties.

PTSD Checklist for DSM-5

The PTSD Checklist for DSM-5 (PCL-5) is a widely used self-report measure used to assess symptoms of post-traumatic stress disorder (PTSD) based on the diagnostic criteria outlined in the fifth edition of the Diagnostic and Statistical Manual of Mental Disorders (DSM-5).

Quantitative Electroencephalography

The Quantitative Electroencephalography (qEEG) is a type of brain imaging analysis that involves the measurement of electrical activity in the brain. Unlike traditional electroencephalography (EEG), which records brain wave activity in a qualitative manner, qEEG provides a quantitative analysis of the data. This allows for a more detailed assessment of brain wave patterns, including the frequency, amplitude, and distribution of electrical activity across different regions of the brain. In clinical settings, qEEG has been employed to aid in the diagnosis and treatment planning for conditions such as epilepsy, ADHD, and other neurological and psychiatric disorders.

SCAN-3 Tests for Auditory Processing Disorders

The SCAN-3 Test for Auditory Processing Disorders (SCAN-3:C for children) and (SCAN-3:A for adults) is an assessment tool used to evaluate individuals for auditory processing disorders (APD). APD refers to difficulties in processing and interpreting auditory information, even though the person's hearing may be normal.

SSP Behavioral Symptoms Pre- and Post-Test

The SSP Behavioral Symptoms Pre- and Post-Test is used to evaluate changes in behavioral symptoms before and after undergoing the SSP intervention. Participants or their caregivers are asked to provide information about symptoms, such as hypersensitivities, communication challenges, emotional dysregulation, attention difficulties, and social engagement issues. The assessment helps track progress and provides valuable information for treatment planning, monitoring outcomes, and making adjustments to the intervention if needed.

SSP Intake Form

The SSP Intake Form is a document used to initiate a conversation about the client. It collects information about the individual's history, sensory sensitivities, autonomic tendencies, home environment, access to supportive people and resources, upcoming stressful experiences, and their specific concerns or goals related to participating in SSP. Not an assessment per se, the SSP Intake Form is the start of an autonomic conversation between the provider and client.

Appendix 2

Short- and Long-Term Effects of Autonomic Dysregulation on Various Bodily Systems

Cardiovascular System

- Short term: Changes in heart rate, blood pressure, and blood vessel dilation may result in symptoms such as palpitations, lightheadedness, dizziness, or fainting

- Long term: Orthostatic intolerance (difficulty maintaining blood pressure when changing positions), tachycardia (persistent elevated heart rate), high blood pressure, and dysautonomia

Respiratory System

- Short term: Breathing patterns may be affected, changing respiratory rate and depth and causing rapid or shallow breathing

- Long term: Dyspnea (shortness of breath/gasping for air), hyperventilation syndrome

Gastrointestinal System

- Short term: Disruptions in digestion may lead to nausea, abdominal pain, bloating, constipation, and diarrhea

- Long term: Dysmotility, or impaired movement of the digestive tract, leading potentially to gastroparesis or irritable bowel syndrome

Metabolic Function

- Short term: Impacts on energy metabolism and the balance of glucose and insulin in the bloodstream

- Long term: Metabolic disorders, insulin resistance, high blood pressure

Temperature Regulation

- Short term: Disruptions in temperature regulation, leading to sensations of overheating or excessive sweating

- Long term: Hypothermia and hyperthermia, which could lead to organ failure

Musculoskeletal System

- Short term: Changes in muscle tone and tension can occur, contributing to symptoms such as muscle stiffness, pain, or tremors

- Long term: Myofascial pain syndrome, chronic pain syndrome

Endocrine System

- Short term: Hormonal imbalance affecting metabolism, sexual function, reproduction, disruption of sleep-wake cycle, and mood

- Long term: Infertility, diabetes, thyroid disease, sexual dysfunction, obesity, depression, anxiety

Immune System

- Short term: Disruption of immune response, potentially impacting susceptibility to infection or autoimmune conditions

- Long term: Autoimmune disorders, increased risk of cancer, damage to the heart, lungs, nervous system or digestive tract

Cognitive Function

- Short term: Brain fog, poor access to executive functions leading to difficulties with concentration, memory, and impulse control

- Long term: Impulsivity, lack of motivation, fatigue, insomnia, mood disturbances

Emotional and Mental Health

- Short term: Mood swings, anger outbursts, anxiety, depression, disrupted sleep patterns, difficulty connecting with others

- Long term: Major depressive disorder, insomnia, panic attacks, chronic loneliness, self-harming behaviors, eating disorders, substance abuse

Multiple Systems

- Short term: Decreased energy, fatigue, inflammation, frequent illness, frequent headaches

- Long term: Chronic fatigue, fibromyalgia, multiple chemical sensitivity, functional neurological disorders, noncardiac chest pain, chronic pelvic pain, chronic inflammatory diseases

Appendix 3

Personalized Regulation Toolboxes

Create your own personalized Regulation Toolbox as described in chapter 4 by adding favorite activities and personalized descriptions of your autonomic states.

VENTRAL VAGAL REGULATION TOOLBOX

Recognize Your Physiological State

Draw your own icon

Metaphor:

Description:

Color:

Create Awareness of Your Physical Sensations

Acknowledge Your Thoughts, Emotions, and Behaviors

Activities for Regulation in a Ventral Vagal State

SYMPATHETIC REGULATION TOOLBOX

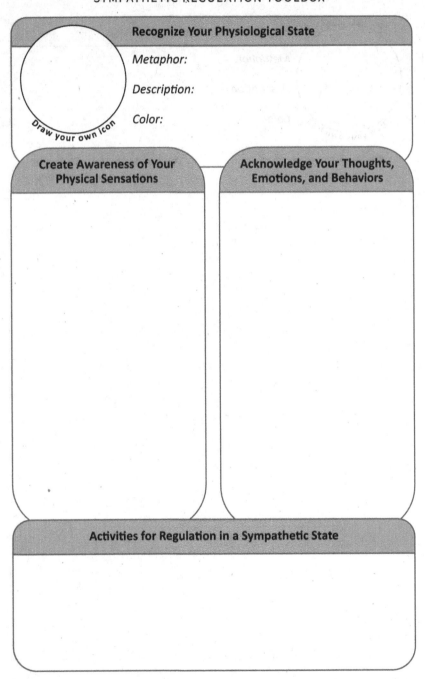

Recognize Your Physiological State

Metaphor:

Description:

Color:

Draw your own icon

Create Awareness of Your Physical Sensations

Acknowledge Your Thoughts, Emotions, and Behaviors

Activities for Regulation in a Sympathetic State

DORSAL VAGAL REGULATION TOOLBOX

Recognize Your Physiological State

Draw your own icon

Metaphor:

Description:

Color:

Create Awareness of Your Physical Sensations

Acknowledge Your Thoughts, Emotions, and Behaviors

Activities for Regulation in a Dorsal Vagal State

Appendix 4

Polyvagal Insights

The following polyvagal insights illustrate PVT in action. By viewing the world through a polyvagal lens, we gain a more compassionate and optimistic perspective on our lives and how we live them. Polyvagal insights highlight the influence of safety or threat in all areas of life and relationships. These influences are evident in our own behaviors and those of others, offering valuable perspectives and guidance in areas like parenting, teaching, medicine, employee development, coaching, therapy, and essentially any human interaction.

In each case story, these insights are denoted in footnotes, identifying the specific polyvagal insights as they appear.

Polyvagal Insight 1: Autonomic State Functions as an Intervening Variable

Autonomic state serves as a platform for our thoughts, feelings, and behaviors, acting as an intervening variable between the world and our response to it. Unlike traditional learning models that focus on stimulus-response associations, PVT emphasizes the role of autonomic state in shaping these associations and frames how we interpret situations and respond. Our autonomic state can increase or decrease our reactivity to events and stimuli thereby framing the same events or stimuli with a different story.

For example, in a dorsal vagal shutdown state, an event may cause feelings of overwhelm and withdrawal. In an activated sympathetic state, it might cause anxiety and agitation. However, in a ventral vagal state, the very same event can evoke curiosity and openness, and even a potentially negative stimulus may not be upsetting.

Through a polyvagal lens, our responses and behaviors are not intentional or shaped by rewards and punishments. Instead, they are part of an adaptive, reflexive system wired into our nervous system, influencing our thoughts, feelings, and behaviors beyond our full voluntary control.

Understanding this helps us develop greater self-awareness and cultivate empathy for others' behaviors. Recognizing the impact of our autonomic states can help interrupt a downward spiral and even initiate an upward one.

When we feel safe, our nervous system is primed to interpret interactions positively, leading to improved communication, reduced misunderstandings, and greater empathy and compassion.

Polyvagal Insight 2: Autonomic States Bias Our Feelings, Thoughts, and Behaviors

Although described as distinct, autonomic states exist on a continuum, subtly influencing our sensations, emotions, thoughts, and behaviors.

In a ventral vagal state, we feel a sense of welcome, connection, and creativity. Blended states like play, flow, quiet connection, and intimacy incorporate the SES. When threats arise, defensive states are triggered. A sympathetic state brings increased activation and hypervigilance, often hindering authentic connection and executive functioning. Blended states involving sympathetic input include play, flow, productivity, and freeze. In a dorsal vagal state, individuals may experience overwhelm, numbness, and shutdown. Blended states with dorsal vagal input are moments of quiet connection and intimacy, rest and restoration, and freeze.

Cues of safety from our surroundings, relationships, and SSP help the ANS reengage in a ventral vagal state, supporting homeostatic functions and fostering greater calm and connection. This state enhances our emotional regulation and ability to navigate social interactions while also helping us understand the nuances of our states and tendencies. As a result, we can communicate more effectively, anticipate our needs, and take better care of ourselves.

Polyvagal Insight 3: Neuroception Detects Cues of Threat and Safety and Alters Autonomic State

Neuroception operates swiftly and unconsciously, detecting cues of safety, danger, or life threat from internal, external, or relational sources. This reflexive process instantaneously shifts autonomic states to support adaptive survival responses. While we may not consciously perceive the inputs to neuroception, we do notice its outputs through bodily changes like shifts in heart rate, breathing, and muscle tension.

Shaped by life experiences, neuroception can sometimes lead us to detect threats where none exist or overlook real dangers. Accurate detection and interpretation of neuroception are crucial for our survival and well-being.

Awareness of our neuroception empowers us to make informed choices. By structuring our environment with more cues of safety and minimizing situations and people that trigger a neuroception of threat, we can enhance our overall sense of security.

Polyvagal Insight 4: The Power of Social Connection and Co-Regulation

Social connection and co-regulation are fundamental human needs, essential for our health and well-being. Co-regulation, facilitated by the activation of the SES, involves a mutually regulating interaction where both individuals feel valued, heard, and in sync.

The cues exchanged between individuals—such as eye contact, facial expressivity, and vocal tone—are reciprocal, influencing and regulating the nervous systems of both parties. Cultivating co-regulating relationships fosters feelings of safety and connection, which, in turn, enhance our ability to develop self-regulation skills. When we feel safe, we can engage socially, forming new connections and deepening existing relationships.

The ability to regulate another's nervous system alongside our own through co-regulation provides invaluable support during times of stress. This cultivates emotional resilience, deepens trust, and allows for the de-escalation of difficult situations, promoting collaboration. As a result, we become better communicators and feel more understood and connected.

Polyvagal Insight 5: Autonomic State Impacts Social Cues

Our nonverbal social cues broadcast our current autonomic state, reflecting how we feel internally and influencing our interactions with others. The five cranial nerves of the SES work together to coordinate the tone and tempo of our voice, eye contact, facial expressions, auditory processing, head and neck movements, and heart rate regulation.

These nonverbal cues can change significantly depending on our autonomic state. In defensive states, expressivity often diminishes, facial tension increases, and our voice may become louder, higher or lower in pitch, or monotone. We might also shake our head or avert our gaze, signaling disagreement or disinterest. Conversely, in a ventral vagal state, these cues soften, becoming more open, warm, modulated, and relaxed.

Not only do our social cues reflect our own autonomic state, but they can also influence the autonomic state of others.

Polyvagal Insight 6: Autonomic State, Vocal Intonation, and Middle Ear Muscle Regulation Mutually Influence Each Other

The mutual influences among autonomic state, intonation of voice, and the regulation of our capacity for auditory perception has broad implications.

In states of threat, our middle ear muscles loosen and prioritize low and high frequencies associated with danger, potentially keeping us locked in a state of threat. Defensive states will also affect the quality of our voice, shifting it to have less prosody and be higher pitched, signaling distress. In a ventral vagal state, those muscles tighten, dampening low frequencies and enhancing the perception of human voices. Our own voice becomes warmer, more melodic, and modulated, conveying ease and engagement.

Our soundscape and the voices of people we spend time with will affect our state. And our state will also affect what we can hear and what we tune out.

Polyvagal Insight 7: The ANS Can Be Retuned to Prioritize Connection and Well-Being

The brain naturally forms and strengthens neuronal connections through neuroplasticity as new concepts are learned. Similarly, the brainstem's regulation of the ANS is neuroplastic, allowing for autonomic responses to be retuned.

Practices in self-regulation, like SSP and other modalities that emphasize the brain-body connection, can enhance this ability for change. Transitioning repeatedly from a defensive state to a connected, ventral vagal one enhances autonomic resilience. By flexibly and appropriately shifting along the continuum of autonomic states, we increase our access to social connection and overall well-being.

Polyvagal Insight 8: The ANS Is at the Core of Our Physical and Mental Wellness

Our physical and mental health thrive when our ANS is in a state of safety, which optimizes homeostatic processes that support healing and recovery.

The brain, nervous system, and visceral organs are interconnected through bidirectional neural pathways, enabling dynamic regulation and maintaining homeostasis. This interconnectedness highlights the ANS's central role in physiological and psychological well-being, as most symptoms and ailments are both physical and mental.

Chronic defensiveness disrupts these homeostatic processes, leading to inflammation and reduced vagal tone. Conditions such as irritable bowel syndrome, fibromyalgia, heart disease, diabetes, and depression can be linked to these disruptions.

To improve health, regulating the stressed nervous system through co-regulation and therapeutic approaches that enhance homeostasis is helpful. With appropriate interventions, the nervous system can support the body's natural healing processes, promote overall health, and foster hope and resilience.

Glossary

afferent nerve pathways: Afferent nerves are sensory fibers that send information from the visceral organs and tissues to the brain. Approximately 80 to 90 percent of the signals sent via the vagus nerve are afferent.

ANS: An abbreviation for *autonomic nervous system.*

auditory hypersensitivities: Heightened sensitivity or responses to sounds that are experienced as pain or discomfort, while not bothersome to most.

autonomic nervous system (ANS): A division of the peripheral nervous system that regulates involuntary bodily functions such as heart rate, respiratory rate, blood pressure, pupillary response, digestion, urination, and sexual function. The ANS comprises three branches—sympathetic, parasympathetic, and enteric—that work together to maintain homeostasis and support health, growth, and restoration. Polyvagal Theory emphasizes the sympathetic and parasympathetic components.

autonomic state: Also known as physiological state. Refers to the current condition of the body's involuntary functions. According to Polyvagal Theory (PVT), there are three primary states: ventral vagal, sympathetic, and dorsal vagal. These states respectively support social connection, activation for fight/flight responses, or immobilized defensive behaviors. PVT assumes an "expanded" autonomic nervous system that appreciates the integration of autonomic pathways with other bodily physiological processes including endocrine, immune, and neuropeptide processes. Thus, the terms *autonomic state* and *physiological state* are used interchangeably in this book.

autonomic tendency: The natural inclination or predisposition to reflexively shift to a specific autonomic state in response to challenges, including danger cues. Some individuals tend to move to a sympathetic or dorsal vagal state, while others may exhibit a hybrid defensive state, such as the cyclic defense loop.

brainstem: A vital part of the brain and a key intersection between the brain and bodily organs involved in essential survival functions such as breathing, heart rate, blood pressure, respiration, and swallowing. Relevant to Safe and Sound Protocol, within the brainstem, the ventral vagal complex integrates both afferent (sensory/feeling) signals from the body and efferent (motor/behavior) signals from higher brain regions to coordinate ventral vagal output and corresponding autonomic, social, and emotional responses.

complex trauma: A condition resulting from exposure to multiple traumatic events over time, typically beginning in childhood. This exposure can disrupt the normal development of the brain and nervous system, impacting emotional regulation, relationships, and overall functioning.

co-regulation: The harmonious relationship between individuals that enables the mutual regulation of autonomic states. Through the social engagement system, one person's nervous system can influence another's, promoting both emotional and physiological well-being.

cranial nerves (CNs): A bundle of nerve fibers that transmits electrical impulses. There are 12 pairs of CNs originating from the brain and extending into various parts of the body. These nerves support a wide range of functions, including sensory perception (such as vision, hearing, taste, and smell), movement of the head and neck muscles, and autonomic functions like regulating heart rate, breathing, and digestion.

Dan Siegel's Hand Model of the Brain: A simplified metaphor for describing brain structure. In this model, the palm represents the brainstem, essential for basic bodily functions. The thumb—folded into the palm—symbolizes the limbic system, which regulates emotions and memory. The fingers, folded over the thumb, depict the cerebral cortex responsible for higher cognition and complex thought processes. When calm, the fingers rest on the thumb allowing clear thinking and sound decision-making. However, under stress, the fingers lift ("flipping our lid"), illustrating a disconnect between rational thought and emotions.

developmental trauma: Developmental trauma refers to adverse experiences during critical periods of childhood development that disrupt healthy growth and have long-term effects on an individual's physical and emotional well-being. Unlike a single traumatic event, developmental trauma involves pervasive exposure to stressful or harmful conditions during the formative years of a person's life. It can dysregulate the autonomic nervous system, affect attachment, impair cognition, and increase vulnerability to stress and trauma throughout the lifespan. With appropriate therapeutic interventions, it is possible to heal from developmental trauma.

diaphragm: A dome-shaped muscle that spans from the bottom of the rib cage, separating the chest cavity from the abdominal cavity. It plays a crucial role in breathing: when you inhale, the diaphragm contracts and moves downward, allowing the lungs to fill with air. During exhalation, it relaxes and moves upward, helping to expel air from the lungs.

dissociation: A phenomenon during which a person experiences a disconnection from their experiences, thoughts, feelings, or sense of identity. Often a coping mechanism in response to trauma, it can create a buffer from painful experiences. Dissociation exists on a continuum, ranging from mild detachment, such as daydreaming, to severe interruption in conscious experience. Through the lens of Polyvagal Theory, dissociation is an adaptive response to a prolonged neuroception of life threat.

dorsal vagal state: An autonomic state supporting immobilized defensive behaviors such as shutdown due to a neuroception of life threat. However, when integrated with the social engagement system it contributes to an immobilization state without fear that is highlighted in shared moments of intimacy.

dysregulation: Difficulty maintaining homeostasis in the autonomic nervous system, resulting in imbalances in both emotional and physiological responses. A dysregulated nervous system remains in a persistent state of threat leading to manifestations such as mood swings, impulsivity, anxiety, social withdrawal, and hypervigilance and physical symptoms like chronic pain, gastrointestinal problems, fatigue, and other related effects.

efferent nerve pathways: Neural pathways also known as motor fibers that transmit signals from the brain to tissues and organs. They control skeletal motor functions and regulate visceral organ activities. Approximately 10 to 20 percent of the signals carried by the vagus nerve are efferent.

heart rate variability (HRV): Heart rate variability is a measure of the variation in the time intervals between each heartbeat. It reflects the neural and nonneural influences on the sinoatrial node, the heart's pacemaker. Higher HRV suggests greater neural regulation of the heart, indicating that the autonomic nervous system is more adept at managing stress and maintaining health. Conversely, lower HRV often indicates a reduced neural regulation, which may signal stress or health challenges.

hertz (Hz): A unit measuring the number of sound wave cycles per second. Humans with excellent hearing typically hear sounds from 20 Hz to 20,000 Hz with lower frequencies perceived as bass and higher frequencies as treble.

implicit memory: Long-term memories acquired unconsciously, often without awareness and sometimes pre-verbally. These memories can influence thoughts and behaviors at a later time.

insula: A region of the brain in the cerebral cortex that integrates information from the body and facilitates communication among different brain regions. It plays a crucial role in interoception, receiving signals from the body and organs and integrating this information with emotional and cognitive processes.

interoception: The process of being aware of and sensing one's internal bodily sensations and condition. Interoception allows for conscious awareness of the body's internal state and plays a role in perceiving safety or threat through neuroception.

middle ear muscles: Two small muscles—the tensor tympani and the stapedius—located in the middle ear that play an important role in auditory processing. Influenced by the facial and trigeminal nerves (two of the five cranial nerves associated with the ventral vagal complex), these muscles control the tension of the eardrum by tightening to dampen background noise to enhance the perception of speech or relaxing to prioritize low and high frequencies associated with threats. The coordination of the activity of these muscles is often influenced by autonomic state. Safe and Sound Protocol was engineered to recruit the neural regulation of the middle ear muscles.

myelinated vs. unmyelinated pathways: Two types of nerve fibers in the nervous system differentiated by the presence or absence of a protective fatty coating of neuronal connections called myelin. Myelinated pathways are covered with myelin, allowing for faster transmission of nerve signals. The ventral vagus nerve is predominantly myelinated, while the dorsal vagus is primarily composed of unmyelinated fibers.

neural exercise: A practice or approach designed to stimulate change and improve brain and nervous system function.

neural feedback loops: Bidirectional circuits of neurons that allow the nervous system to communicate and regulate mental and physical responses to internal and external stimuli.

neural pathways: Bundles of nerve fibers that establish connections among neurons within and between various regions of the nervous system. These routes of connection form complex networks that enable sensory perception, motor control, cognitive functions, and the regulation of bodily processes.

neural regulation: The set of mechanisms and processes by which the nervous system controls and coordinates physical and cognitive functions in response to internal and external stimuli. Fundamental to many aspects of functioning, it includes integrating sensory information, processing signals, and activating appropriate responses to maintain homeostasis and adapt to changing conditions.

neuroception: The neural evaluation of safety and threat that reflexively triggers shifts in autonomic state without requiring conscious awareness. Not to be confused with perception and interoception, which both require awareness.

neuromodulator: A substance or input that modulates or influences the activity of the nervous system. A neuromodulator acts broadly to regulate the overall activity of neural circuits. For example, electrical stimulation of the vagus as well as social engagement and co-regulation are neuromodulators of autonomic state.

nucleus ambiguus: A brainstem region located within the ventral vagal complex from which the myelinated ventral vagus nerve originates.

perseverative thinking: Repetitive or prolonged thought patterns that involve repeatedly revisiting or dwelling on events, often without resolution. Perseverative thinking can include rumination, where individuals get stuck replaying past events or problems, leading to impaired concentration and increased anxiety and affecting overall well-being.

physiological state: See autonomic state.

Polyvagal Theory (PVT): A theory that explains how the autonomic nervous system regulates our physiological state and affects our behavior. Often referred to as the science of safety, PVT posits that our physiological state forms the foundation for our sensations, thoughts, emotions, and behaviors.

prosody: The rhythm, intonation, and variations in pitch, volume, and tempo in speech that convey meaning beyond the words spoken. Prosody communicates emotions, emphasis, and nuances in speech, significantly influencing how listeners interpret spoken language.

In general, prosody tends to be used to describe the positive affect embedded in speech.

PVT: An abbreviation for *Polyvagal Theory.*

regulation: In the context of the autonomic nervous system, regulation refers to the system's ability to maintain balance (homeostasis) and flexibility (resilience) in various mental and physical functions. Regulating one's autonomic state involves balancing the influences of sympathetic and parasympathetic states to sustain optimal physiological and emotional equilibrium, as well as adaptability.

retained primitive reflexes: Primitive reflexes are involuntary, automatic movements present at birth that are critical for a baby's development. When these reflexes persist beyond the developmental period, they are considered "retained" and can indicate developmental delays or neurodevelopmental issues.

Safe and Sound Protocol (SSP): A noninvasive therapy based on Polyvagal Theory, SSP involves listening to music that has been filtered to prioritize the frequencies of human speech. This auditory input enables the nervous system to be receptive to cues of safety and to downregulate defensiveness.

self-regulation: An individual's ability to manage their thoughts, emotions, and behaviors from a well-balanced autonomic nervous system. Self-regulation develops through co-regulation and can be strengthened by ongoing reciprocal social interactions with others. Self-regulation practices refer to activities that enhance the capacity for self-regulation when co-regulation is not possible.

shock trauma: A severe physical or psychological injury from a sudden, overwhelming event such as a severe accident, natural disaster, or violent assault. It can manifest as extreme physical and psychological pain, often accompanied by shock.

social engagement system (SES): A neural network involving five cranial nerves that enables individuals to detect and respond to social cues, thereby fostering positive social interactions. Activation of the SES occurs through ventral vagal outflow, facilitating pro-social signals such as facial expressions, vocalizations, listening acuity, head tilting, and regulation of the heart and lungs. This activation supports social connection by promoting engagement.

SSP: An abbreviation for *Safe and Sound Protocol*.

sympathetic state: An autonomic state supporting mobilized defensive behaviors, such as fight or flight, due to a neuroception of threat or danger.

vagal brake: A metaphor describing the capacity of the vagus nerve to slow heart rate when safety is perceived through neuroception. Physiologically, this is achieved through the release of acetylcholine. The metaphor extends to "releasing the vagal brake" to allow for a higher heart rate, increasing physiological activation to meet threats or engage in activities such as exercise, mental effort, and even simple movements. Vagal efficiency quantifies the effectiveness of the vagal brake.

vagal efficiency (VE): A specific measure of the robustness of the vagal brake quantified by the relationship between cardiac vagal tone (measured by respiratory sinus arrhythmia) and heart rate. Higher VE is associated with better access to the social engagement system. It also indicates more efficient regulation of heart rate, reflecting one's ability to respond effectively to stressors and maintain homeostasis. Lower VE seems to be an index of a dysregulated autonomic nervous.

vagal tone: The activity of the vagus nerve measured through the amplitude of respiratory sinus arrhythmia, a component of heart rate variability characterized by the rhythmic increases and decreases in heart rate within the frequency band of spontaneous breathing. It reflects the influence of the vagus nerve on heart rate regulation and is enhanced by experiences that support social and emotional engagement.

vagus nerve: The 10th cranial nerve and the longest and most complex of the 12 cranial nerves. Extending from the brainstem through the neck and into the abdomen, it plays a fundamental role in the autonomic nervous system by regulating various involuntary bodily functions. Through its afferent (sensory) and efferent (motor) pathways, the vagus nerve helps maintain psychological and physiological homeostasis.

ventral vagal state: An autonomic state dependent on the ventral vagal complex that supports social engagement behaviors like cooperation and connection. A neuroception of safety automatically moves the individual into a ventral vagal state.

viscera: Our internal organs such as the heart, lungs, digestive organs (stomach, intestines, etc.), liver, kidneys, and other vital organs.

Notes

Introduction: Retuning the Autonomic Nervous System to Generate Change and Connection

1. Stephen W. Porges, "Orienting in a Defensive World: Mammalian Modifications of Our Evolutionary Heritage; A Polyvagal Theory," *Psychophysiology* 32, no. 4 (1995): 301–18; Stephen W. Porges, "The Vagal Paradox: A Polyvagal Solution," *Comprehensive Psychoneuroendocrinology* 16 (2023): 100200, doi.org/10.1016/j.cpnec.2023.100200.

2. Porges, "Orienting"; Porges, "Vagal Paradox."

3. Eugene T. Gendlin, *Experiencing and the Creation of Meaning: A Philosophical and Psychological Approach to the Subjective* (Evanston, IL: Northwestern University Press, 1997).

Chapter 1: The Autonomic Nervous System Through the Lens of Polyvagal Theory

1. Stephen W. Porges, "Polyvagal Theory: A Science of Safety," *Frontiers in Integrative Neuroscience* 16 (2022): 871227, doi.org/10.3389/fnint.2022.871227.

2. K. J. Mahler, *Interoception: The Eighth Sensory System* (Shawnee Mission, KS: AAPC Publishing, 2015).

3. R. Bailey et al., "Appeasement: Replacing Stockholm Syndrome as a Definition of a Survival Strategy," *European Journal of Psychotraumatology* 14, no. 1 (2023): 2161038, doi.org/10.1080/20008066.2022.2161038.

4. Deb Dana, *Anchored: How to Befriend Your Nervous System Using Polyvagal Theory* (Boulder, CO: Sounds True, 2021).

Chapter 2: The Safe and Sound Protocol: A Groundbreaking Polyvagal Approach

1. U.S. surgeon general, *Our Epidemic of Loneliness and Isolation: The U.S. Surgeon General's Advisory on the Healing Effects of Social Connection and Community* (Government Printing Office, 2023).
2. Theodosius Dobzhansky (1900–1975). Exact wording may be a paraphrase or adaptation.
3. Stephen W. Porges, "Polyvagal Theory: A Science of Safety," *Frontiers in Integrative Neuroscience* 16 (2022): 871227, doi.org/10.3389/fnint.2022.871227.
4. Oliver Sacks, *Musicophilia: Tales of Music and the Brain* (New York: Vintage, 2007).
5. Martina de Witte et al., "Music Therapy for Stress Reduction: A Systematic Review and Meta-Analysis," *Health Psychology Review* 16, no.1 (2020): 134-159, doi.org/10.1080/17437199.2020.1846580.
6. Robert Gupta, an American violinist and physician, has expressed this sentiment in various talks and interviews, highlighting the intersection of music and healing.
7. Graham F. Welch et al., "Editorial: The Impact of Music on Human Development and Well-Being," *Frontiers in Psychology* 11 (2020): 1246, doi.org/10.3389/fpsyg.2020.01246.
8. Stephen W. Porges et al., "Respiratory Sinus Arrhythmia and Auditory Processing in Autism: Modifiable Deficits of an Integrated Social Engagement System?" *International Journal of Psychophysiology* 88, no. 3 (2013): 261–70.
9. Deb Dana, *Polyvagal Exercises for Safety and Connection* (New York: W. W. Norton & Company, 2020), 47–50.
10. K. Kovacic et al., "Impaired Vagal Efficiency Predicts Auricular Neurostimulation Response in Adolescent Functional Abdominal Pain Disorders," *The American Journal of Gastroenterology* 115, no. 9 (2020): 1534–38.

11. Porges et al., "Respiratory Sinus Arrhythmia," 261–70.

12. Stephen W. Porges et al., "Reducing Auditory Hypersensitivities in Autistic Spectrum Disorder: Preliminary Findings Evaluating the Listening Project Protocol," *Frontiers in Pediatrics* 2 (2014): 80.

13. Keri J. Heilman et al., "Effects of the Safe and Sound Protocol (SSP) on Sensory Processing, Digestive Function, and Selective Eating in Children and Adults with Autism: A Prospective Single-Arm Study," *Journal on Developmental Disabilities* 28, no. 1 (2023): 1–26.

14. Heleen Grooten-Bresser et al., "Effects of Safe and Sound Protocol on Self-Reported Autonomic Reactivity, Anxiety, and Depression in Speech Therapy Clients with Voice, Throat, and Breathing Complaints," *Music and Medicine: An Interdisciplinary Journal* 16, no. 2 (2024).

15. C. Hawkes et al., "Neuromodulation Using Computer-Altered Music to Treat a Ten-Year-Old Child Unresponsive to Standard Interventions for Functional Neurological Disorder," *Harvard Review of Psychiatry* 30, no. 5 (2022): 303–16, doi.org/10.1097/HRP.0000000000000341.

16. J. Kolacz et al., "Frequency Filtered Music in Trauma Therapy: Results from a Controlled Trial" (paper presented at the International Society for Traumatic Stress Studies Annual Meeting, Los Angeles, CA, November 2023).

Chapter 3: How the Safe and Sound Protocol Works

1. J. Kolacz, Gregory F. Lewis, and Stephen W. Porges, "The Integration of Vocal Communication and Biobehavioral State Regulation in Mammals: A Polyvagal Hypothesis," in *Handbook of Behavioral Neuroscience*, ed. Stanislaw M. Brudzynski, vol. 25 (Amsterdam: Elsevier, 2018), 23–34.

2. Ilona Poćwierz-Marciniak and Michał Harciarek, "The Effect of Musical Stimulation and Mother's Voice on the Early Development of Musical Abilities: A Neuropsychological Perspective," *International Journal of Environmental Research and Public Health* 18, no. 16 (2021): 8467.

3. J. Kolacz et al., "Associations Between Acoustic Features of Maternal Speech and Infants' Emotion Regulation Following a Social Stressor," *Infancy: The Official Journal of the International Society on Infant Studies* 27, no. 1 (2022): 135–58, doi.org/10.1111/infa.12440.

4. Erik Borg and Stephen A. Counter, "The Middle-Ear Muscles," *Scientific American* 261, no. 2 (1989): 74.

5. Kevin J. Tracey, "The Inflammatory Reflex," *Nature* 420, no. 6917 (2002): 853–59, doi.org/10.1038/nature01321.

Chapter 4: Self-Directed Change and Healing: Retuning the Nervous System

1. Bethany E. Kok and Barbara L. Fredrickson, "Upward Spirals of the Heart: Autonomic Flexibility, as Indexed by Vagal Tone, Reciprocally and Prospectively Predicts Positive Emotions and Social Connectedness," *Biological Psychology* 85, no. 3 (2010): 432–36, doi.org/10.1016/j.biopsycho.2010.09.005.

2. William James, *Habit* (New York: H. Holt and Company, 1914).

3. Valentin Magnon, Frédéric Dutheil, and Guillaume T. Vallet, "Benefits from One Session of Deep and Slow Breathing on Vagal Tone and Anxiety in Young and Older Adults," *Scientific Reports* 11, no. 19267 (2021), doi.org/10.1038/s41598-021-98736-9; X. Ma et al., "The Effect of Diaphragmatic Breathing on Attention, Negative Affect, and Stress in Healthy Adults," *Frontiers in Psychology* 8 (2017): 874, doi.org/10.3389/fpsyg.2017.00874.

4. Stanley Rosenberg, *Accessing the Healing Power of the Vagus Nerve: Self-Help Exercises for Anxiety, Depression, Trauma, and Autism* (Berkeley: North Atlantic Books, 2017).

5. Resources for Resilience (R4R) is a project of the Association for Comprehensive Energy Psychology's (ACEP) Humanitarian Committee. Members from all over the world volunteer their time to meet R4R's mission and provide free access to self-help techniques that can help you recover more quickly and easily from stressful events. The full set of resources can be found at r4r .energypsych.org.

6. Soothing Butterfly Hug, originated and developed by Lucina Artigas, Resources for Resilience, r4r.energypsych.org/finding-safety-and -connection.

7. Havening Techniques, developed by Ron Ruden, Resources for Resilience, r4r.energypsych.org/finding-safety-and-connection.

8. Healing Head Hold, adapted from Terrence Bennett's Touch for Health neuro/vascular points, Resources for Resilience, r4r .energypsych.org/calming-and-balancing.

9. Cross Crawl/Crossover Shoulder Pull, developed by Paul and Gail Dennison and Donna Eden, Resources for Resilience, r4r .energypsych.org/clearing-confusion-and-clumsiness.

10. Linda Chamberlain, *Howling with Huskies: And Other Ways to Feel Good!* (Victoria, BC, Canada: Tellwell Talent, 2022).

Chapter 6: Hannah Rediscovers Her Voice and Vitality

1. Heleen Grooten-Bresser et al., "Effects of Safe and Sound Protocol on Self-Reported Autonomic Reactivity, Anxiety, and Depression in Speech Therapy Clients with Voice, Throat, and Breathing Complaints," *Music and Medicine: An Interdisciplinary Journal* 16, no. 2 (2024).

2. F. Jadhakhan et al., "Prevalence of Medically Unexplained Symptoms in Adults Who Are High Users of Healthcare Services and Magnitude of Associated Costs: A Systematic Review," *BMJ Open* 12, no. 10 (2022): e059971, doi.org/10.1136/bmjopen-2021-059971.

Chapter 7: From Chronic Pain and Hearing Loss to Healing, Hope, and Joy

1. Walter R. Hess, "The Central Control of the Activity of Internal Organs" (Nobel Lecture, presented on December 12, 1949), nobelprize.org/prizes/medicine/1949/hess/lecture/.

2. Walter Cannon, *The Wisdom of the Body* (New York: W. W. Norton & Company, 1932).

3. Claude Bernard, *An Introduction to the Study of Experimental Medicine*, trans. Henry Copley Greene (New York: Dover Publications, 1957), 121–23.

4. Roland Staud, "Heart Rate Variability as a Biomarker of Fibromyalgia Syndrome," *Future Rheumatology* 3, no. 5 (2008): 475–83; Nazar Mazurak et al., "Heart Rate Variability in the Irritable Bowel Syndrome: A Review of the Literature," *Neurogastroenterology and Motility* 24, no. 3 (2012): 206–16.

Chapter 8: Tormented Teen Gets Her Life Back

1. U.S. Centers for Disease Control and Prevention, High School Youth Risk Behavior Survey, cdc.gov/healthyyouth/data/yrbs/overview .htm.

2. Stephen W. Porges, "Orienting in a Defensive World: Mammalian Modification of Our Evolutionary Heritage. A Polyvagal Theory," *Psychophysiology* 32, no. 4 (1995): 301–18.

3. J. Kolacz et al., "Associations Between Acoustic Features of Maternal Speech and Infants' Emotion Regulation Following a Social Stressor," *Infancy: The Official Journal of the International Society on Infant Studies* 27, no. 1 (2022): 135–58, doi.org/10.1111/infa.12440.

4. Hope Peterson et al., "The Sober Salience Network: Exploring the Link Between Vagal Efficiency and Brain Network Topology During Alcohol Image Viewing Following Abstinence," SSRN, 2023, ssrn .com/abstract=4438356 or dx.doi.org/10.2139/ssrn.4438356.

5. R. L. Johnson and C. G. Wilson, "A Review of Vagus Nerve Stimulation as a Therapeutic Intervention," *Journal of Inflammation Research* 11 (2018): 203–13, doi.org/10.2147/JIR.S163248.

Chapter 9: Uwase's Recovery from Disabling Dissociation

1. J. Kolacz et al., "Sexual Function in Adults with a History of Childhood Maltreatment: Mediating Effects of Self-Reported Autonomic Reactivity," *Psychological Trauma: Theory, Research, Practice, and Policy* 12, no. 3 (2020): 281–90; J. Kolacz et al.,

"Adversity History Predicts Self-Reported Autonomic Reactivity and Mental Health in US Residents During the COVID-19 Pandemic," *Frontiers in Psychiatry* 11 (2020): 1119.

2. Jacek Kolacz et al., "Association of Self-Reported Autonomic Symptoms with Sensor-Based Physiological Measures," *Psychosomatic Medicine* 85, no. 9 (2023): 785–94, doi.org/10.1097 /PSY.0000000000001250.

3. Edward B. Blanchard et al., "Psychometric Properties of the PTSD Checklist (PCL)," *Behavior Research & Therapy* 34, no. 8 (1996): 669–73, doi.org/10.1016/0005-7967(96)00033-2.

4. Ruth Lanius and Ruth Buczynski, "Rethinking Trauma: How Neuroscience Can Give Us a Clearer Picture of Trauma Treatment," NICABM, accessed August 1, 2024, s3.amazonaws.com/nicabm -stealthseminar/Rethinking-trauma-new/Ruth/NICABM -RuthLanius-Transcript.pdf.

Chapter 11: Shifting from Perfectionism to Being "Perfectly Imperfect"

1. Hope Peterson et al., "The Sober Salience Network: Exploring the Link between Vagal Efficiency and Brain Network Topology During Alcohol Image Viewing Following Abstinence," SSRN, 2023, ssrn.com/abstract=4438356 or dx.doi.org/10.2139/ssrn .4438356.

Chapter 12: From Surviving to Thriving with Parkinson's Disease

1. Betsy Polatin, *Humanual (A Manual for Being Human): An Epic Journey to Your Expanded Self* (Cardiff-by-the-Sea, CA: Waterside Productions, 2020).

2. G. Park and J. F. Thayer, "From the Heart to the Mind: Cardiac Vagal Tone Modulates Top-Down and Bottom-Up Visual Perception and Attention to Emotional Stimuli," *Frontiers in Psychology* 5 (2014): 278, doi.org/10.3389/fpsyg.2014.00278.

Chapter 13: Navigating Gender Identity and Selective Mutism

1. K. J. Heilman et al., "Sluggish Vagal Brake Reactivity to Physical Exercise Challenge in Children with Selective Mutism," *Development and Psychopathology* 24, no. 1 (2012): 241–50.

Chapter 14: Unexpected SSP Response Alters the Clinical Arc of Recovery

1. The SEGAN approach is also described in the case study in chapter 10 titled "A Family Heals from Shock and Grief."
2. Thalia Harmony, "The Functional Significance of Delta Oscillations in Cognitive Processing," *Frontiers in Integrative Neuroscience* 7 (2013): 83, doi.org/10.3389/fnint.2013.00083.
3. X. Jia and A. Kohn, "Gamma Rhythms in the Brain," *PLoS Biology* 9, no. 4 (2011): e1001045, doi.org/10.1371/journal.pbio.1001045.
4. P. Sabu et al., "A Review of the Role of Affective Stimuli in Event-Related Frontal Alpha Asymmetry," *Frontiers in Computer Science* 4 (2022), doi.org/10.3389/fcomp.2022.869123.
5. A. Maffei et al., "EEG Alpha Band Functional Connectivity Reveals Distinct Cortical Dynamics for Overt and Covert Emotional Face Processing," *Scientific Reports* 13 (2023): 9951, doi.org/10.1038/s41598-023-36860-4.
6. N. J. Kelley et al., "The Relationship of Approach/Avoidance Motivation and Asymmetric Frontal Cortical Activity: A Review of Studies Manipulating Frontal Asymmetry," *International Journal of Psychophysiology* 119 (2017): 19–30, doi.org/10.1016/j.ijpsycho.2017.03.001.
7. Stephen W. Porges et al., "Respiratory Sinus Arrhythmia and Auditory Processing in Autism: Modifiable Deficits of an Integrated Social Engagement System?" *International Journal of Psychophysiology* 88, no. 3 (2013): 261–70.
8. J. Winhall and S. W. Porges, "Revolutionizing Addiction Treatment with the Felt Sense Polyvagal Model$_{TM}$," *International Body Psychotherapy Journal* 21, no. 1 (2022).

Chapter 15: COVID Recovery and a Renewed Relationship with Self

1. H. E. Davis et al., "Long COVID: Major Findings, Mechanisms and Recommendations," *Nature Reviews Microbiology* 21 (2023), doi.org/10.1038/s41579-022-00846-2.
2. Eric Azabou et al., "Vagus Nerve Stimulation: A Potential Adjunct Therapy for COVID-19," *Frontiers in Medicine* 8 (2021), doi.org/10.3389/fmed.2021.625836.

Chapter 16: From Exclusion to Empowerment: A Boy's Journey with Hypermobility Spectrum Disorder

1. D. Dana, *The Polyvagal Theory in Therapy* (New York: W. W. Norton & Company, 2018), 58–65.
2. T. Ruiz Maya et al., "Dysautonomia in Hypermobile Ehlers-Danlos Syndrome and Hypermobility Spectrum Disorders Is Associated with Exercise Intolerance and Cardiac Atrophy," *American Journal of Medical Genetics Part A* 185, no. 12 (2021): 3754–61, doi.org/10.1002/ajmg.a.62446.

Chapter 17: The Importance of "Being" Rather Than "Doing" as an SSP Provider

1. In their book, *Nourishing Resilience: Helping Clients Move Forward from Developmental Trauma*, Kathy Kain, PhD, and Steve Terrell, PsyD, refer to "foundational dysregulation" as what happens when access to safety is so lacking in early life that dysregulation becomes pervasive and sets the foundation for the development of a person as a whole. Foundational regulation is the result of a sufficient experience of feeling safety, connection, and belonging in the world in early life so that a person can develop the capacity to return to a state of calm presence.
2. Paula is the co-developer, along with Rachel Lewis-Marlow, of the Embodied Recovery Institute, a model for working simultaneously with attachment, defense, and sensory processing. A core feature of this approach is the neurocellular movement patterns from Bonnie

Bainbridge Cohen's Body-Mind Centering. Paula has also studied the work of Dianne Poole Heller, Pat Ogden, Dan Siegel, and Janina Fisher in her understanding of attachment.

3. Thomas Hübl, *Attuned: Practicing Interdependence to Heal Our Trauma—and Our World* (Boulder, CO: Sounds True, 2023).

4. See note 2 for this chapter.

Appendix I: Assessment Descriptions

1. J. C. Sánchez-Manso, R. Gujarathi, and M. Varacallo, "Autonomic Dysfunction," StatPearls, updated August 4, 2023, ncbi.nlm.nih .gov/books/NBK430888/.

Bibliography

Bonaz, Bruno, Valérie Sinniger, and Sonia Pellissier. "Anti-Inflammatory Properties of the Vagus Nerve: Potential Therapeutic Implications of Vagus Nerve Stimulation." *The Journal of Physiology* 594, no. 20 (2016): 5781–90. doi.org/10.1113/JP271539.

Cohen, Bonnie Bainbridge. *Basic Neurocellular Patterns: Exploring Developmental Movement.* El Sobrante, CA: Burchfield Rose Publishers, 2018.

Harricharan, Sharna, Margaret C. McKinnon, and Ruth A. Lanius. "How Processing of Sensory Information from the Internal and External Worlds Shape the Perception and Engagement with the World in the Aftermath of Trauma: Implications for PTSD." *Frontiers in Neuroscience* 15 (2021): 625490. doi.org/10.3389/fnins.2021.625490.

Hübl, Thomas. *Attuned: Practicing Interdependence to Heal Our Trauma—and Our World.* Boulder, CO: Sounds True, 2023.

Kain, Kathy, PhD, and Steve Terrell, PsyD. *Nourishing Resilience: Helping Clients Move Forward from Developmental Trauma.* Berkeley, CA: North Atlantic Books, 2018.

Kolacz, Jacek, Elizabeth B. daSilva, Gregory F. Lewis, Betty I. Bertenthal, and Stephen W. Porges. "Associations Between Acoustic Features of Maternal Speech and Infants' Emotion Regulation Following a Social Stressor." *Infancy: The Official Journal of the International Society on Infant Studies* 27, no. 1 (2022): 135–58. doi.org/10.1111/infa.12440.

Kolacz, Jacek, Gregory F. Lewis, and Stephen W. Porges. "The Integration of Vocal Communication and Biobehavioral State Regulation in Mammals: A Polyvagal Hypothesis." In *Handbook of Behavioral Neuroscience*, vol. 25, 23–34. Amsterdam: Elsevier, 2018.

Namkung, Ho, Sun-Hong Kim, and Akira Sawa. "The Insula: An Underestimated Brain Area in Clinical Neuroscience, Psychiatry, and Neurology." *Trends in Neurosciences* 40, no. 4 (2017): 200–07. doi.org/10.1016/j.tins.2017.02.002.

Porges, Stephen W. "Orienting in a Defensive World: Mammalian Modifications of Our Evolutionary Heritage; A Polyvagal Theory." *Psychophysiology* 32, no. 4 (1995): 301–18.

———. *Polyvagal Safety: Attachment, Communication, Self-Regulation.* New York: Norton Professional Books, 2021.

———. *The Polyvagal Theory: Neurophysiological Foundations of Emotions, Attachment, Communication, and Self-Regulation.* New York: W. W. Norton & Company, 2011.

———. "The Polyvagal Theory: New Insights into Adaptive Reactions of the Autonomic Nervous System." *Cleveland Clinic Journal of Medicine* 76 (2009): S86. doi.org/10.3949/ccjm.76.s2.17.

———. "Polyvagal Theory: A Science of Safety." *Frontiers in Integrative Neuroscience* 16 (2022): 871227.

———. "Vagal Nerve Stimulation Through the Lens of the Polyvagal Theory: Recruiting Neurophysiological Mechanisms to Dampen Threat Reactions and Promote Homeostatic Functions." In *Vagus Nerve Stimulation*, edited by M. G. Frasch and E. C. Porges. Neuromethods, vol. 205. Humana, New York: 2024.

———. "Vagal Pathways: Portals to Compassion." In *The Oxford Handbook of Compassion Science*, edited by Emma M. Seppälä, Emiliana Simon-Thomas, Stephanie L. Brown, Monica C. Worline, C. Daryl Cameron, and James R. Doty. Oxford: Oxford University Press, 2017.

Porges, Stephen W., Olga V. Bazhenova, Elysa Bal, Nancy Carlson, Yevgeniya Sorokin, Keri J. Heilman, Edwin H. Cook, and Gregory F. Lewis. "Reducing Auditory Hypersensitivities in Autistic

Spectrum Disorder: Preliminary Findings Evaluating the Listening Project Protocol." *Frontiers in Pediatrics* 2 (2014): 80. doi.org/10 .3389/fped.2014.00080.

Sánchez-Manso, Juan Carlos, Rahul Gujarathi, and Matthew Varacallo. "Autonomic Dysfunction." StatPearls. Updated August 4, 2023. ncbi .nlm.nih.gov/books/NBK430888/.

Weinstein, Ann Diamond. *Prenatal Development and Parents' Lived Experiences: How Early Events Shaped Our Psychophysiology and Relationships*. Norton Series on Interpersonal Neurobiology. New York: W. W. Norton & Company, 2016.

Index

chronic illness, 200, 207, 208
  Parkinson's Disease, 197–208
  repeating SSP and, 207
chronic pain, 77, 102, 136, 137–48
co-regulation, 26, 40, 67, 102, 202, 205–6,
    265, 268
  in case studies, 3–4, 125–36, 129, 148
  human-animal interactions, 95
  power of, 287–88
  with SSP provider, 16, 42, 51, 52, 67,
    102, 196, 199–200, 205–6, 263
  ventral vagal state and, 37, 86
cognitive behavioral therapy (CBT), 51,
    233
cognitive functioning, 33, 51, 75–76,
    156–57, 279, 286
  COVID and, 239
Cohen, Bonnie Bainbridge, 257
colors
  dorsal vagal state (gray), 34, 88
  sympathetic state (red), 33, 87
  ventral vagal state (green), 33, 86
complex trauma, 125–36, 172
connection, 39–40, 46–47, 183, 241–42
  brain and body, 52, 121, 289
  connected states, 32–33, 34–35, 36
  See also social connection
Corrigan, Frank, 197
cortisol, 25, 33, 47, 77
COVID, 233–42
  acute phase, 235, 239–40
  chronic phase, 239–40
  extreme symptoms, 234–35
  Long COVID, 5–6, 235, 240

social isolation and, 157, 246
  sudden death after, 174
cranial nerves, 27, 67–68
  accessory nerve (XI), 67–68
  facial nerve (VII), 46, 67–68, 70
  glossopharyngeal nerve (IX), 46, 67–68
  trigeminal nerve (V), 46, 67–68, 70
  vagus nerve (X), 27–30, 67–68
Crossover Shoulder Pull, 92
cues of safety, 11, 30, 41, 121–23, 158,
    286
cyclic defense loop, 37–38, 103, 198–99
  case study, 149–60
  gender dysphoria and, 218

Dan Siegel's Hand Model of the Brain,
    247, 292–93
Dana, Deb, 94–95
danger. See threats
death, unexpected, 173–84
Deep Brain Reorienting (DBR), 233, 238
defensive states, 33–34, 37–38, 157–58,
    288
  continuum of, 192–94
  cyclic defense loop, 37–38, 103, 149–
    60, 198–99
  metabolic demands of, 217
  neuropeptides and, 77
defensiveness, 24–25, 26–27, 182
  chronic, 25, 218, 219, 231, 289
  perfectionism and, 192–94
  physiological responses, 33
depression, 46, 59–61, 63, 215
  assessments of, 62, 274, 275

expectations, 188

exploring activities, 85

eye contact, 65, 133, 241

    gaze aversion, 8, 241, 244, 288

eye movement desensitization and
    reprocessing (EMDR), 161, 163,
    168, 170, 178

    combined with SSP, 233, 236

eye muscles, 89, 94

face/facial affect, 197, 198–99, 202, 206

facial nerve (CN VII), 46, 67–68, 70

fainting, 138, 145

fatigue, 152, 252, 279

fawning, 37

feedback

    feedback loops, 68, 80–81, 157, 207,
    254

    neurofeedback, 223, 234, 236

Felt Sense Polyvagal Grounding Practice,
    94

fibromyalgia, 133, 138, 145, 279

fight-or-flight response, 27, 33, 35

fingers (holding your fingers), 93

flashbacks, 4–5, 163, 178

    EMDR for, 178

flat facial affect, 197, 198–99, 202, 206

flexibility, 29, 38, 45, 142–43, 268

    neural exercise and, 41–42, 54, 66, 72

flipping out metaphor, 33, 87

floating metaphor, 33, 86

flopping down metaphor, 34, 88

Frederickson, Barbara, 80–81

freeze state, 36, 128, 210

functional freeze, 256

frequencies. *See* sound frequencies

gastrointestinal issues, 120, 252, 278

gaze aversion, 8, 241, 244, 288

gender dysphoria, 210, 218–19, 220

gender identity, 209–20

glimmers, 94–95

globus pharyngeus, 125, 126, 134

glossopharyngeal nerve (CN IX), 46,
    67–68

Goeltz, Donnalea Van Vleet, 89, 95

gravity, 94

Gray, Amber Elizabeth, 94

grief, 180–81, 184

    case study, 173–84

    rituals and, 176–77, 183–84

Grooten, Heleen, 125–36

hallucinations, 149, 153, 159

Hand-on-Heart, 90–91

Head Hold, 92

healing, 79–95, 101, 289–90

    medically unexplained symptoms,
    102–3

    modalities of, 79, 80

    safety, importance in, 79–80

    upward spirals, 80–81, 102

    See also case studies

Healing Head Hold, 92

hearing, 56–57, 73–74, 157–59, 202

    auditory hypersensitivity, 58–59, 149,
    157–59, 202

    ear infections and, 71, 146

About the Authors

Stephen W. Porges

Stephen W. Porges, PhD, has been an academic for more than 50 years and currently holds positions as a distinguished university scientist at Indiana University, professor of psychiatry at the University of North Carolina and the University of Florida College of Medicine in Jacksonville, and professor emeritus at the University of Illinois at Chicago and the University of Maryland. He has published more than 400 peer-reviewed scientific papers that have been cited in more than 58,000 peer-reviewed papers, and he holds several patents related to technologies involved in monitoring and regulating autonomic state.

Stephen also served as president of the Society for Psychophysiological Research and the Federation of Associations in Behavioral & Brain Sciences and is a former recipient of a National Institute of Mental Health Research Scientist Development Award. He is the originator of the Polyvagal Theory, which emphasizes the importance of physiological state in the expression of behavioral, mental, and health problems, and he is the creator of a music-based intervention, the Safe and Sound Protocol, which is the focus of this book. In collaboration with Anthony Gorry, he cocreated an acoustic intervention, the Rest and Restore Protocol, engineered to support homeostatic functions, and with Karen Onderko, Deb Dana, and Randall Redfield, he founded the Polyvagal Institute.

Karen Onderko

Karen Onderko is committed to advancing the understanding of the nervous system through Polyvagal Theory to enhance therapeutic care and foster greater connection and acceptance among individuals. She was instrumental in transitioning Dr. Porges's Safe and Sound Protocol from the research laboratory into practical, widespread use as an accessible tool now available to therapists across various disciplines worldwide.

Karen was the director of research and education for Integrated Listening Systems and Unyte Health and is a cofounder and current board member of the Polyvagal Institute. She serves on the board of directors for Developmental FX and has served as a board member for Aspen Brain Institute, Denver Film Society, Colorado Academy, and Stanley British Primary School. Before her work in neuroscience, she spent the first half of her career specializing in financial risk management, teaching the use of derivatives to international and central bankers, marketing financial products to banks and corporations, and managing an options business to ensure the safety of retirement investments. Karen holds a degree from Georgetown University and lives in Denver, Colorado, with her husband and three daughters.

About Sounds True

S ounds True was founded in 1985 by Tami Simon with a clear mission: to disseminate spiritual wisdom. Since starting out as a project with one woman and her tape recorder, we have grown into a multimedia publishing company with a catalog of more than 3,000 titles by some of the leading teachers and visionaries of our time, and an ever-expanding family of beloved customers from across the world.

In more than three decades of evolution, Sounds True has maintained our focus on our overriding purpose and mission: to wake up the world. We offer books, audio programs, online learning experiences, and in-person events to support your personal growth and awakening, and to unlock our greatest human capacities to love and serve.

At SoundsTrue.com you'll find a wealth of resources to enrich your journey, including our weekly *Insights at the Edge* podcast, free downloads, and information about our nonprofit Sounds True Foundation, where we strive to remove financial barriers to the materials we publish through scholarships and donations worldwide.

To learn more, please visit SoundsTrue.com/freegifts or call us toll-free at 800.333.9185.

Together, we can wake up the world.

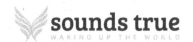